Contents

Who has been kidnapped?   **1**

Preface   **3**

Why did I smoke? Why quit smoking?   **5**

Part 1 Mask of cigarettes

The reason why cigarettes can accompany you through every day is that you choose cigarettes.   **14**

Quitting smoking is like falling out of love. When love disappears, let go bravely.   **18**

Reason 1: The taste of cigarettes is great.   **22**

Reason 2: Smoking can increase self-confidence and sense taste.   **29**

Reason 3: Cigarettes help to relax.   **35**

Reason 4: Smoking makes the stool smoother.   **42**

Reason 5: There is no sense of security without carrying cigarettes on.   **47**

Part 1 QUIZ   **53**

Part 2 Firm determination

Strengthen your beliefs   **56**

Never use any substitutes to help you quit smoking   **65**

N. O. P. E., Not One Puff Ever   **70**

Eliminate Cravings Breathing Method   **74**

Part 2 QUIZ   **79**

Part 3 A new milestone

A new milestone: I started to quit smoking! **81**

The first stage, smoking cessation Day 1 ~ Day 3: Day 1 **85**

The first stage, smoking cessation Day 1 ~ Day 3: Day 2 **90**

The first stage, smoking cessation Day 1 ~ Day 3: Day 3 **94**

The second stage, smoking cessation Day 4 ~ Day 7:
Week 1 **98**

The third stage, smoking cessation Week 2 ~ Week 4:
Month 1 **101**

Finish Line: Congratulations on completing the third stage of quitting smoking. Now you can tell everyone loudly: Yeah, I am a non-smoking person. **105**

Who has been kidnapped?

This book is about how a daily smoker becomes a non-smoker.

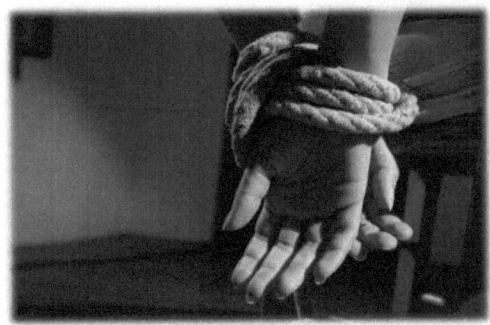

(Only you can break free from shackles. But first, you need to realize the existence of restraints.)

I am the one who had been kidnapped for 20 years, in other words, I was the victim. But before I got rid of the addiction, I never thought someone had kidnapped me.

I thought that everything was voluntary. After all, I smoked my first cigarette, right?

Although I know all the disadvantages of smoking, whenever someone told me about the defects of smoking and to quit smoking, I defended cigarettes. This is like the Stockholm syndrome, the hostages defended the kidnappers and even fell in love with the kidnappers. So, unless you break away from tobacco addiction, you're probably defending cigarettes now, aren't you?

Before I became a non-smoker, I thought I couldn't live without cigarettes all my life. It's like:

Many people think that quitting smoking is impossible.
Many people think it's hard to quit smoking.
Many people have never thought about quitting smoking.

But the facts are:

As early as a hundred years ago, people thought that flying was impossible.
Fifty years ago, people also found it was difficult to land on the moon.
Now, the hardest thing you've done is to find the book, as for quitting smoking, it is much easier.

You don't have to stop smoking right now and you don't have to agree with me. But if you think smoking **MAKES SENSE**, then this book should be able to help you quit smoking.

Preface

Please take out a cigarette and light it. While you are smoking, please feel it:

Do you enjoy smoking? What does smoking make you feel?
Does it relax you, help you concentrate, make you increase self-confidence...? Or just because you enjoy the taste of cigarettes

◎ **This book can't get you to quit smoking unless you want to.**
◎ **I'm not going to teach you how to quit smoking. I'm just going to tell you some details that are easily overlooked by smokers and what would happen when you quit smoking.**
◎ **You are the one who bravely quit smoking, not me.**
◎ **You are the winner, not me.**

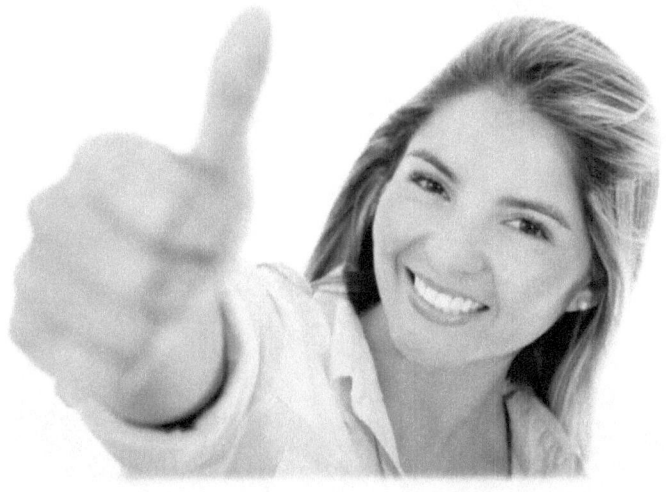

Now, have you finished your cigarette?

If you have finished smoking, it is a perfect time to look back on the reason why you want smoking:

Do you still think cigarettes taste good?
Do you still feel relaxed?
Have you become more confident?

If not, why smoke?

(Quitting smoking, since the last time you extinguished the cigarette, it started quietly)

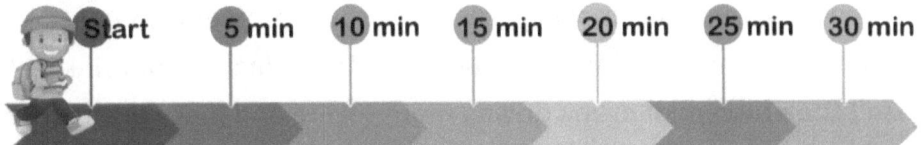

Start   5 min   10 min   15 min   20 min   25 min   30 min

Why did I smoke? Why quit smoking?

Before giving up smoking, I had smoked for twenty years.

I never felt smoking cigarettes is bad. Although smoking was harmful to my health, it made me feel good. I used to say that if a person does not have a good mood, how can he have a healthy body?

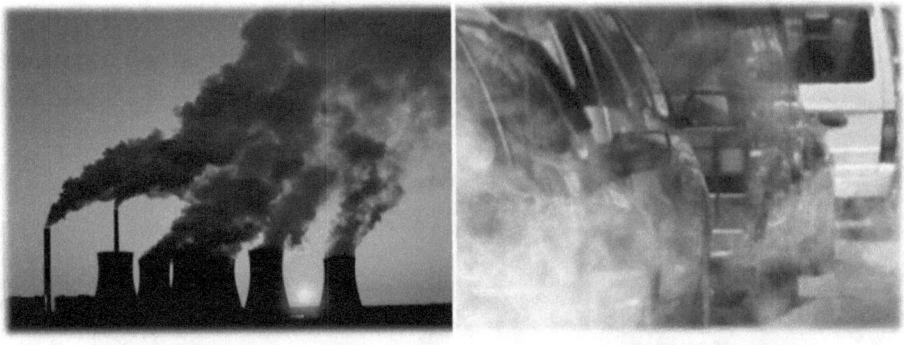

(The pollution caused by power plants and vehicles.)

Smoking causes air pollution? If so, isn't the pollution caused by the waste gases from thermal power plants, industrial pollution and old vehicles more serious?

Somebody says that smoking can create social problems that cigarettes are a stepping stone for drug users. What about drinking? Isn't the problem of drunk driving more severe and more destructive to society?

I smoke two packs of cigarettes a day. Once I hospitalized because of pneumonia, I felt chest pain when I breathed, but even so, I still smoked. After discharged from the hospital, my family found that I still coughed a lot and asked me to quit smoking. But I told them that it was caused by nose allergy, had nothing to do with cigarettes, even if I quit smoking, I would still cough.

I was single during those years. My friend introduced me to a nurse who hated the smell of cigarettes very much. I tried not to smoke in front of her, but it was useless. For a non-smoker, the smell of smoke was very easy to sniff out.

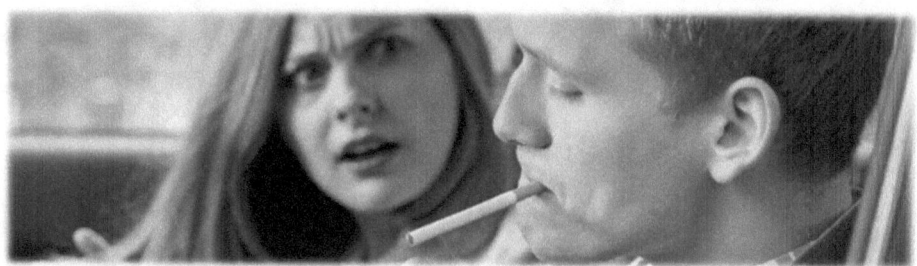

(The non-smokers are sensitive to the smell of cigarettes.)

Once we went to the movies. For a guy who smokes every half hour, watching movies is such a painful thing. I kept running out to smoke, and I didn't even know what the movie was about. After the show, the nurse said to me: Can't you bear to smoke for 2 hours and concentrate on a movie? I replied: Why should I hold back?

Since that time, we have never contacted again.

I didn't know why I should quit smoking. I thought it was a pleasant thing to smoke, and I didn't think it has any terrible effect on my health. Even if someone asked me if I had ever tried to quit smoking, I would say: Although I haven't tried to quit smoking, yet, it should be easy, the only matter is if I want to do it or not.

So, day after day, and after a long time, I got married. Until one day, my wife said to me: Hubby, have you been upset lately? Why smoke more and more?

My wife never asked me to quit smoking. She thought that smoking was a habit that existed before I met her. Although it was not a good thing, it was also part of me.

She told me that if I quit smoking, she would be very happy for me. It doesn't matter if I don't want to quit smoking, but don't smoke too much. After all, excessive smoking is bad for my health.

I tried to reduce the number of cigarettes to one pack a day, but it didn't seem as simple as I thought. Every time I wanted to cut the numbers, I smoked more the next day. It made me feel like there's a devil's advocate in my body, singing a different tune. The more I want to remove it, the tighter it bites.

In this way, I began to think seriously:

Why do I smoke more and more?
Why on earth do I smoke?
What am I insisting or defending?

In the past, I was on the same line with cigarettes. I rationalized smoking and found out many reasons why it was necessary to smoke. For example, I used to smoke before going to stool every day, and I would have the feeling of defecation. Otherwise, even if I sat on the toilet for a whole day, I couldn't solve the bowel movement. I must smoke a cigarette after every meal so that I can feel satisfied. Before I gave a speech, I must smoke a cigarette. Smoking could help me make my mind organized. I also liked the taste of tobacco. With only sniffing it or with one puff, I could tell you what brand of cigarettes it is.

However, whenever I refused to smoke, tried to push cigarettes away but failed and been pulled back by cigarettes, the more I see the essence: What I thought that I liked smoking, I needed to smoke, smoking was necessary, was just my brain that made it up to rationalize smoking addiction. Before I became addicted to cigarettes, I didn't have the habits of smoking when doing certain things. There had never been a problem of not being able to do something without smoking, or any regrets or losses in my life without cigarettes.

Then, I have to admit that I am rebellious, because in the past, anyone who advised me to quit smoking, I would think he was the one who gave me a hard time. But when cigarettes continued to pull me, I began to think: Who is the biggest profiteer from my smoking?

The cigarette addiction that grips me tightly, like a blood-sucking worm, which I can't get rid of, who is the manipulator behind it? The cigarette company, isn't it? Yes, but in addition to the cigarette companies, there's another one behind the scenes: The government.

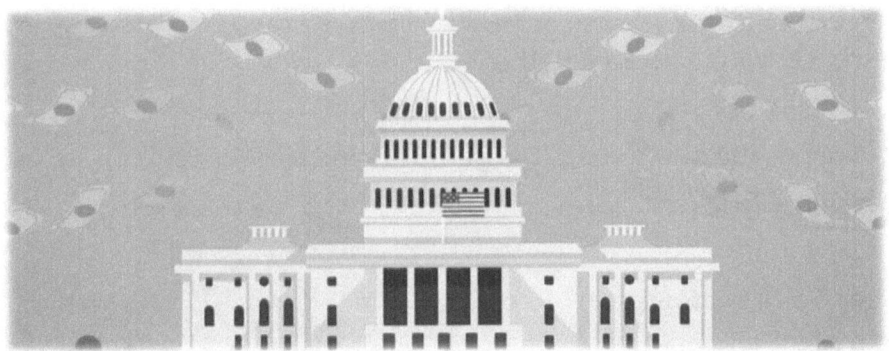

(The government is the biggest beneficiary.)

The profits of cigarettes are astonishing. A pack of cigarettes, about 20% of the price, is the profit of the cigarette company; but more than half of the price is paid to the government. The government using various names such as welfare, health benefits, etc., levies heavy taxes on smokers. But these taxes are not used to benefit smokers. The government spends a small amount of tax to promote anti-smoking, but it doesn't spend the money on the construction of smoking zones in public areas, so that smokers can smoke in fixed locations in different sections of the road, with good separations between smokers and non-smokers.

The government describes smokers as polluters, continually increasing the tax on cigarettes, but not feeding back those taxes to smokers; although the government has been advocating that smoking can cause cancer, heart disease, emphysema and so on, telling everyone not to smoke, but this seems to be only to show the responsibility of good advocacy. As if it had settled on smokers, the government knew they would continue to smoke, and all the price increases would be accepted.

It reminds me of the song "Dangerous" sung by Michael Jackson, in which the lyrics are:

She's So Dangerous
The Girl Is So Dangerous
Take Away My Money
Throw Away My Time
You Can Call Me Honey
But You're No Damn Good For Me

What is the reason for smokers willing to be exploited layer after layer? It is nicotine addiction. Nicotine addiction makes cigarettes become a cash cow for cigarette companies and governments. Once addicted, cigarettes become a dangerous girl in the lyrics. Knowing that cigarettes are dangerous, wasting money and wasting time, although you can get some illusions of happiness, it is useless.

Now, step by step, let's break the myths related to cigarettes. These myths are the excuses I used to refuse to quit smoking, and they are also the parts that many people find difficult to give up when they quit smoking. The longer you smoke, the less you remember the previous "YOU" who did not smoke. From a different perspective, let's look at the temptation of cigarettes at different angles, and perhaps it would be better for us to understand the nature of cigarettes and the black hands hidden behind cigarettes.

Please don't feel like I'm trying to persuade you to quit smoking. I am just sharing the journey of my quitting smoking and some sorts I discovered during the process, that's it.

At any time you read the book, when you hear the call of cigarettes, you can pick up a cigarette and smoke without restraint.
But remember, every time you smoke, it means that you acquiesce the black hands hidden behind the cigarettes to rob you.

On the beginning page of each chapter in this book, you will see a picture like this:

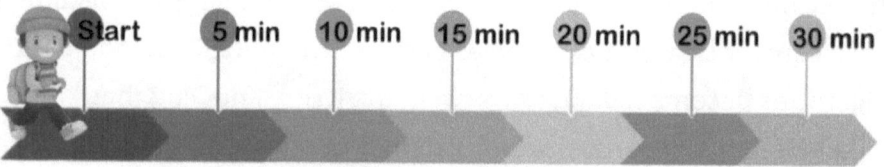

(The timeline of quitting)

This picture shows how much time has passed since the last time you smoked a cigarette. Smokers must know that it is hard to resist smoking when the craving comes. It is hard to accumulate non-smoking hours, but it can be easily destroyed in just five seconds by a puff of cigarettes. Because of this, through the picture reminder, I hope every smoker can cherish his accumulated smoking cessation hours.

You can definitely read this book while smoking, but when you finish smoking, please start reading from the first page of the book again, so that the book can play its maximum role. Of course, this is only a suggestion. It's up to you to decide whether or not to do so.

• Part 1 •

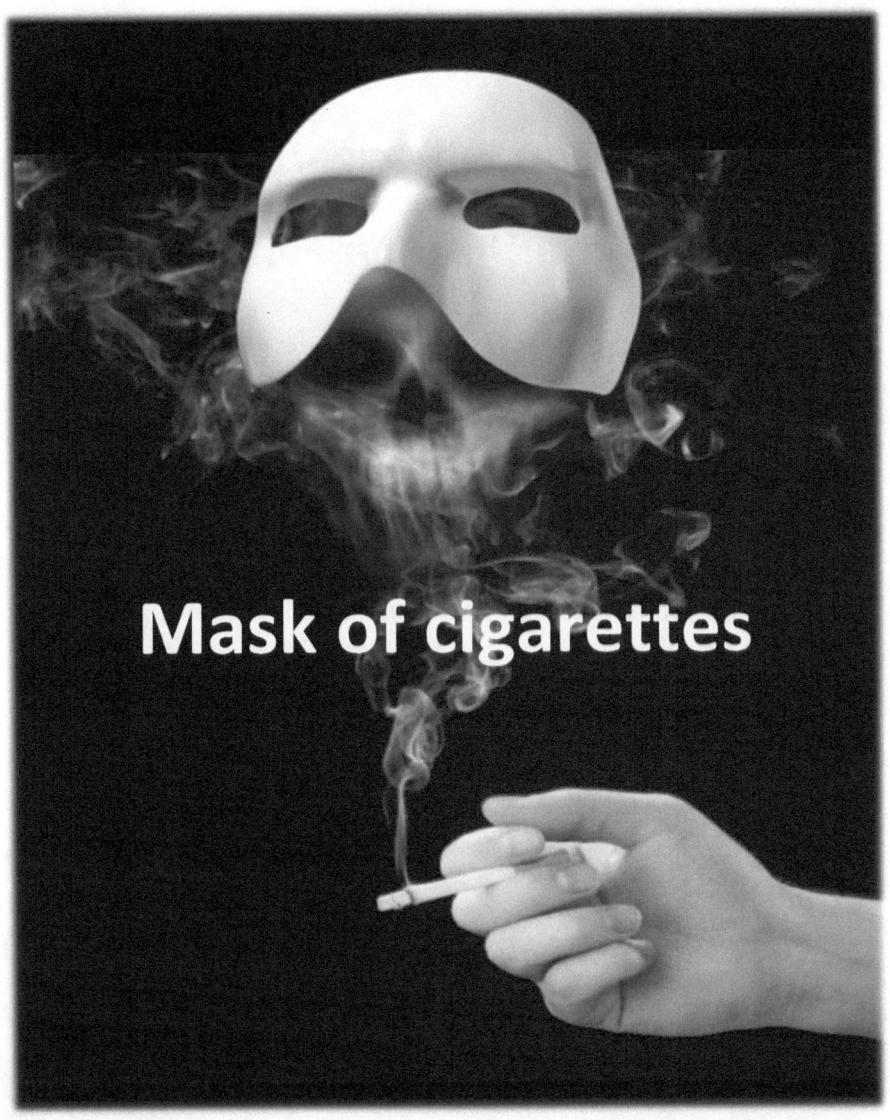

Mask of cigarettes

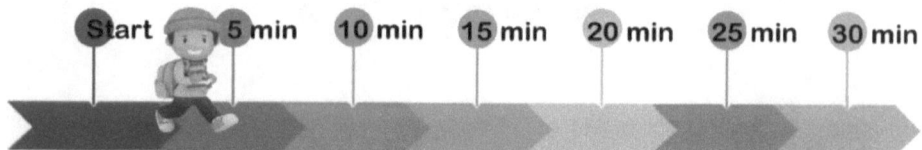

(Success in quitting smoking means not smoking the next cigarette)

Start 5 min 10 min 15 min 20 min 25 min 30 min

The reason why cigarettes can accompany you through every day is that you choose cigarettes.

An old man who had participated in the Vietnam War was coughing while still smoking a cigarette.

Every time he took a cigarette, he coughed a few times, sometimes he coughed too hard so that the breathing seems to be suspended; But when he did not smoke, his breathing was shallower, strictly speaking, he was simply panting.

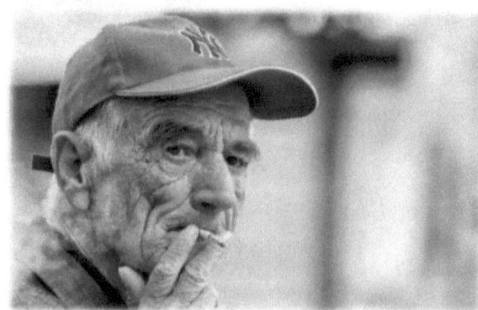

(The old man, Andrew Tripp, told his stories with cigarettes. Even he coughed seriously, he still smoked one after another.)

He held the cigarette with index and middle fingers in his shaking hand; but whenever the hand holding the cigarette closing to the mouth, it stopped shaking magically, so that the lips could catch the filter of the cigarette accurately.

I asked the old man if he had ever thought about quitting smoking. He said, "When I was in Vietnam, the sky was raining, the ground was full of traps covered by leaves, bullets flew by my ears, and shells exploded behind me, killed my companions on the spot. It was a place where even God did not exist. When I was alone in the jungle waiting for a rescue, the only thing that accompanied me was the pack of cigarettes on my helmet."

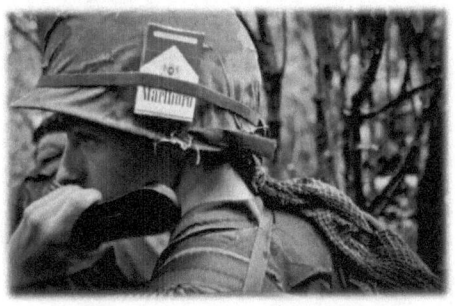

(Cigarettes on the helmet)

Son, you haven't experienced war, have you? You probably not know the feeling of isolation and despair. At that time, the Vietnam Communists searched beside me and almost found me several times. I had planned to pull out the pistol and fought with them if they got me. I prayed to God that even if the jungle battlefield was my place of death, let me smoke the last cigarette before leaving the world. I prayed to God that even if the jungle battlefield was my place of death, let me smoke the last cigarette before leaving the world.

As a result, a miracle happened, the Viet Cong suddenly left. I quickly climbed out of the grass and fled back to the base. When I was safe, the first thing I did was smoking. Now, please tell me: if you were me, would you want to quit smoking?

After I heard the old man told me this story, I got very emotional. I didn't answer his question at the moment. After three months, I went to see the old man again and tried to tell him my answer before I realized that he had passed away. The cause of his death was chronic obstructive pulmonary disease, which is COPD.

I was going to tell him: I am very shocked by your experience, and I am even more respectful and admired. As you said, in such a dangerous situation on the battlefield, the Viet Cong is a deadly enemy. They took the lives of your fellow robes, but they didn't take you away. You survived; On the other hand, in the case of desperation, cigarettes were the only thing that accompanied you, your only hope in such a desperate situation. Now you are in the paradise of freedom. There are no bullets or traps of the Vietcong. But for you, cigarettes are more dangerous than the Vietcong. If you continue to smoke, it will kill you.

Unexpectedly, cigarettes really killed him. O Lord, let perpetual light shine upon him. May the soul of the faithful departed, through the mercy of God, rest in peace.

Every time you light, smoke, and extinguish a cigarette, this process may contain a story. As time goes by, cigarettes seem to be a good companion or spiritual sustenance in your life. But whether it is a partner or a companion, there is a premise: this partner or companion won't harm you. However, cigarettes are not, it hurts your health, and it keeps you spending money.

Some people think that cigarettes are good companions because they carry cigarettes all the time. If you also think that cigarettes are your spiritual sustenance, then from today on, you might as well try something else: If you are a devout Christian, from now on, take the cross with you whenever and wherever you are. Next time, whenever you are nervous, anxious, upset, bored, etc., take the cross out and hold it in your palm, and then practice Smoke-Free Breathing(which will be explained later), and soon you will find that the cross is a better spiritual sustenance than cigarettes.

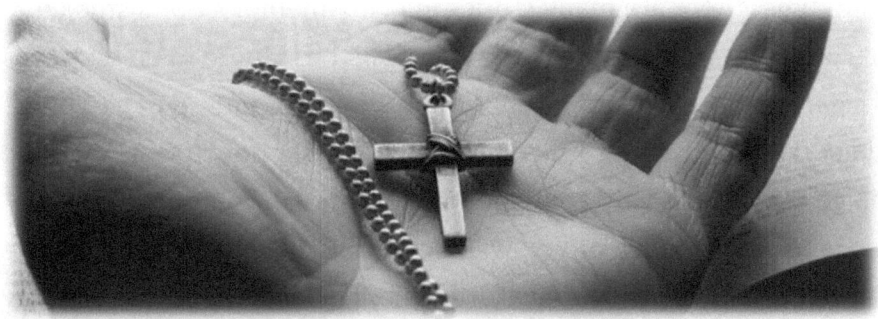

(The cross is definitely a better spiritual support.)

(You can always pick up cigarettes easily, but the accumulated smoking cessation hours turn to zero.)

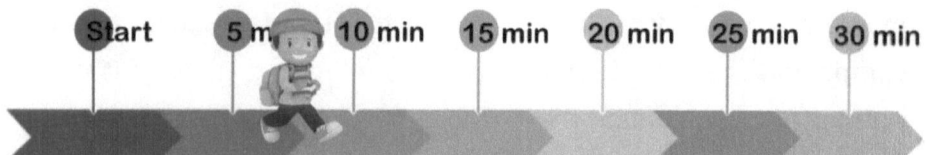

Start   5 min   10 min   15 min   20 min   25 min   30 min

Quitting smoking is like falling out of love. When love disappears, let go bravely.

Y ou won't forget that you used to be addicted to cigarettes, but you choose not to smoke any more.

In life time, there are many stories in every memory. For a smoker, the longer he smokes, the more stories he has. There must be traces of cigarettes in each story. Don't think when you get rid of cigarette addiction after quitting smoking, you will forget how to smoke, or you can go back to the way of life before you smoke, you don't have the desire to smoke at all, or you will forget how to light a cigarette, even you will be choked by the cigarette when you light it... these are totally impossible.

In fact, smoking is like riding a bicycle, once you can ride, even if you haven't ridden for a long time, you won't forget it. So does smoking, no matter how long you have not smoked, just put the cigarette into your mouth and light it, you will know what to do next.

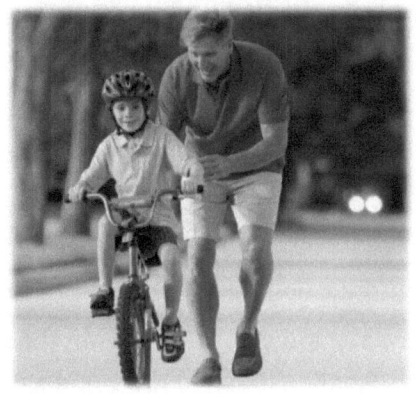

(Smoking is like riding a bike, once you learned how to smoke, you will never forget it.)

Therefore, the so-called quitting smoking means not smoking again. You do know how to light cigarettes, how to mix the smoke with air, and how to breathe in the lungs, these will never be forgotten. But after quitting, unlike the current situation: It is now you want to smoke and you are driven to smoke when you have cravings. But after quitting, you will control yourself and will not smoke again, with or without cravings.

I think it's more appropriate to compare quitting smoking to being lovelorn. Once you quit smoking, it feels like a person you love, suddenly told you that she is in love with somebody else, and then you broke up. Although you still love her, you know breaking up is good for each other, no matter how much you miss her or think about her, you won't go to see her again.

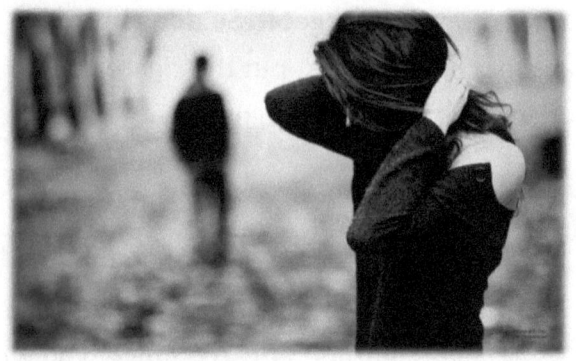

(Quitting smoking is pretty much like ended a relationship, being heartbroken.)

It's hard to live without a loved one. Two people who were inseparable from each other have lived their lives since then. You may think about her all the time during the day, and you can't do anything. Just like lovelorn, when you first quit smoking, you may not want to do anything except smoking in your mind. You are both anxious and depressed, and you feel ants in your pants. You want to pick up a cigarette and smoke, even only a puff, just as you've already said goodbye, but you still want to see her again, even if it's a glance in distance. Your head tells you not to be impulsive when love is past, it is superfluous to get her back just because you can't forget her. Similarly, when the determination to quit smoking has been made, even a small puff will put you back in the previous state.

A few days passed, the torn heart slowed down a little bit, it is no longer so painful, but she will still be remembered at certain moments of the day, especially those moments you had been doing things together. The same is true of quitting smoking, after a few days of stopping smoking, the discomfort situation is significantly less painful than the first few days, but at certain moments of the day, smoking is particularly desirable, sometimes after meals, sometimes after getting up in the morning. These specific periods of cravings won't last long, and they won't be particularly difficult. They will be diverted by some things and will soon be transferred. After all, the most painful stage has passed, and the rest is to maintain the hard-won results.

After another few days, you won't want to smoke for most of your daily life, but if you do something that you don't usually do, such as taking a trip, and you haven't quit smoking yet last time you traveled, the craving may come out again during this situation.

The cravings will become less and weaker over time, and the frequency will be lower and lower, but it will never be forgotten. Even after many years, it will still be remembered. Just like the ex-girlfriend who abandoned you and broke up with you many years ago, now you bump into her on the street, and she keeps telling you that she met someone unkind and want to make up with you, what would you do? You already have your own life, you survived the hardest days yourself, don't make the same mistakes again. Otherwise, the price of insanity is getting stuck in hell.

Next, let's see **what reasons are often used to rationalize smoking**.

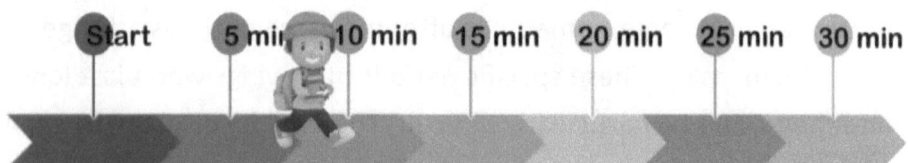

(When the craving comes, focus on how to get through the time.)

Start 5 min 10 min 15 min 20 min 25 min 30 min

Reason 1: The taste of cigarettes is great.

If you still feel that cigarettes smell good or taste delicious in your mouth, especially you have put it out for nearly 10 minutes since you finished your last smoke, and you still feel the taste of cigarettes in your mouth is delicious, you can put this book down because it means you really like cigarettes, and you can tell the reasons why you like them.

But in fact, almost all smokers hate the taste of cigarettes before they become addicted, whether they sniff or taste it. And a smoker, when he quits cigarettes, he will be more sensitive to the taste or smell of cigarettes than an average person.

Please don't get me wrong. I am not denying the taste of cigarettes because of my position. Natural tobacco does have a charming, unique aroma, but it is a natural aroma which is completely different from the burning of tobacco or the taste of a cigarette.

Please try to recall before you became addicted, or when you were still a child, you must also hate the smell of cigarettes.

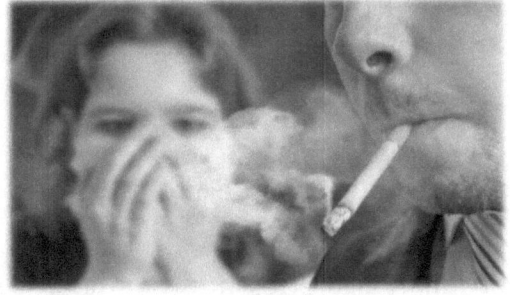

(Only smoker himself doesn't mind the smoke he made.)

If you can't remember, try to stay in an enclosed space with a non-smoking person and smoke your own cigarettes. I promise that person will be crazy. This is not because of the awareness of anti-smoking, or the rejection of second-hand smoking, but it is really choking, smelling like tear gas, it suffocates people.

Or you can try to spit the smoke on a child, a dog, or a cat, and see how they reacted. They are the least deceptive, and they definitely will run away as soon as they smell the smoke.

Someone once told me: But I smoke at home, and my wife and children have never complained about it. If you did the same thing, smoking at home, but your families never complained, then you really owe them a big hug and say sorry to them. Because they really love you, they would rather endure the unpleasant smell of smoke that you made than let you be wronged, or tell you not to smoke at home.

If you change cigarettes into burning straw today and give it to a smoker, do you know what will happen? He will choke to death and cough incessantly until his lungs are coughing out. But for a non-smoker, a bystander, burning straw and burning cigarettes smell no different.

Speaking of the taste of cigarettes, this is even more interesting.

What does it taste like when you inhale cigarettes into your mouth? A bit bitter and spicy, right?

You can do an experiment. After each cigarette is smoked, throw the cigarette butt into a cup filled with water. After a day, you can see the situation of the cup: the water in the cup becomes stinky and black, you never want to drink it.

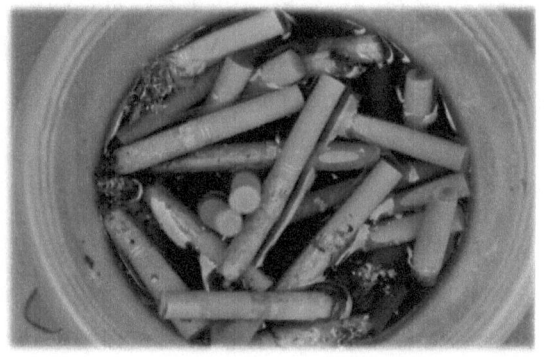

(Is this tasty? You wouldn't even want to smell it, not mention to drink it.)

The reason why it becomes black and smelly is that the tar in the cigarette is released into the water. Tar is a dark brown or black viscous liquid of hydrocarbons and free carbon, obtained from a wide variety of organic materials through destructive distillation. Tar can be produced from coal, wood, petroleum, or peat. Its main use was in preserving wooden sailing vessels against rot. The word "tar" refers primarily to a substance that is derived from the wood and roots of pine. In earlier times it was often used as a water repellent coating for boats, ships, and roofs. Tar can also be used as a medicine for the treatment of certain skin diseases, making mummy, and paving the road.

Although tar is such useful, the advantages and disadvantages of tar are not the focus of discussion. What we want to explore is: Why is it so ugly, you wouldn't eat the tar in your mouth at all, but you would breathe it into your lungs? Isn't there any feeling of nausea? Some people even defend cigarettes and praise them for their good taste, why?

Please don't argue with me about what cigarettes taste in your mouth! As long as a person who has never smoked, whether he is smoking or after he smoked, the taste in his mouth must be bitter and spicy, without any fragrance at all.

Why do some people think that the taste of cigarettes is great? It's all about nicotine, the key ingredient in addiction. When you are smoking, inhaling nicotine stimulates the brain to secrete more dopamine. Some studies have found that nicotine increases the level of dopamine in the brain. Dopamine is a neurotransmitter. It transmits exciting information and is also related to addiction.

So dopamine represents happiness? This is not the case. Studies have shown that the essence of the dopamine reward pathway is getting reward, which is getting feedback, not happiness.

What is the reward? The reward is that after you did it once, you want to do it a second time. In general, we receive substantial feedback, such as an apple, then the apple's taste, touch, and other physical properties are linked to the reward system after conversion to neural information, resulting in synapse production. With the change in plasticity, you know that apples are delicious and go to eat apples.

More studies have found that the effectiveness of dopamine results are from expecting rewards rather than getting rewards. Dopamine brings cravings and fantasies.

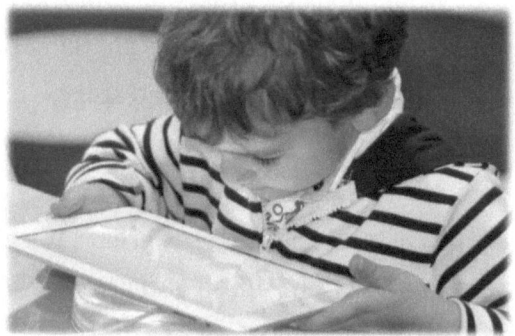

(Being addicted is a kind of feedback that can happen at any age, including children.)

This is like the case of modern people using social media on their mobile phones. Many times, we just keep sliding and click on the "next" message. Even if we are tired, we are reluctant to let go. This is the reward mechanism of dopamine telling you, "The next message will be very exciting." When you force yourself to put down your mobile phone, you will feel very anxious. Dopamine just makes us look forward to the next one. This is an addiction.

Addiction is completely different from contentment and happiness. Even when you use the source of addiction, it only gives you a sense of hunger but does not give you satisfaction. Or, it makes you feel hungrier than satisfaction and then misleads your brain to create contradictions and make wrong judgments.

So smokers don't think the taste of cigarettes in their mouths is spicy and bitter, just because the misjudgment made by the brain? Yes, absolutely right. Because the brain knows that it is a necessity to get nicotine by smoking, to increase dopamine in the brain, and to ease the cravings of tobacco, the brain regards smoking as a reasonable action, so the feeling that against or contradict this behavior is blocked by the brain.

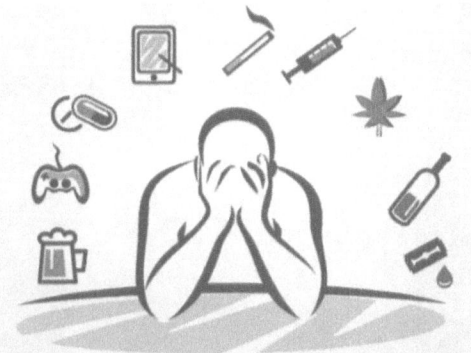

(Many things are addictive, alcohol, pornography, substance abuse, spending sprees, even self-harm.)

This is like a drug addict. When he is in withdraw, he can't feel the pain when he pierces the needle into his skin, in order to achieve the purpose of drug use.

In the same situation, you can also see other things, for example, people who like to drink wine or drink coffee, he can tell you how good wine or coffee is, but cannot feel the spicy taste of the wine or the bitterness of coffee, and the same is true.

(Don't let the withdrawal of cigarettes addiction bother you. Every time you want to smoke, but you don't, it disappears naturally.)

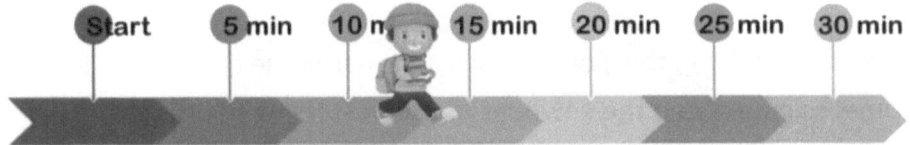

| Start | 5 min | 10 m... | 15 min | 20 min | 25 min | 30 min |

Reason 2: Smoking can increase self-confidence and sense taste.

Seriously, when I first learned to smoke, I really had the feeling that smoking can increase self-confidence. At that time, I lacked

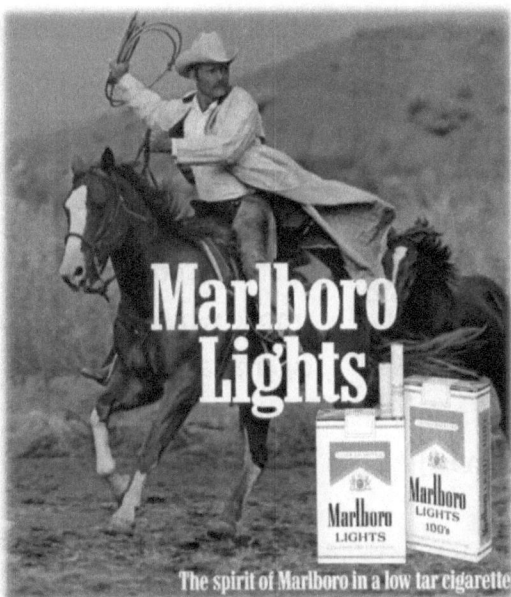

Marlboro Lights

Marlboro LIGHTS

Marlboro LIGHTS 100's

The spirit of Marlboro in a low tar cigarette.

self-confidence. Whenever I had to face the masses or talk to ladies, I had to light up my cigarette and take a few puffs to speak boldly.

(The use of the Marlboro Man campaign had very significant and immediate effects on

sales.)

Frankly speaking, this poster really conquered me completely at that time. I appreciated the cowboys in the posters, who emitted masculinity and boldness. Even then, I always thought that smoking this brand of cigarettes would turn me into the cowboy in the poster. In fact, the first cigarette I smoked was this brand.

Twenty years ago, at the end of the last century, when I first started smoking, most of the places at that time were friendly to smokers and smoking indoors would not be prohibited. Otherwise, smoking and non-smoking areas would be delimited in the same space. The price of cigarettes was also low, and a pack of Marlboro cost only $1.8 US dollars. But do you think that era was a paradise for addicts? If we go

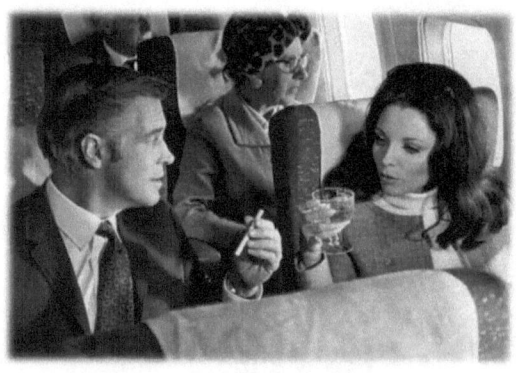

back 20 years, back to the 1980s, teachers could smoke in class, government officials could smoke in meetings, or even passengers could smoke when taking a plane, cigarettes were a part of people's daily life.

(People smoked on planes.)

But things have changed. With the development of science and technology, more and more diseases have been proved to be directly or indirectly related to cigarettes. Most countries have banned smoking indoors in public places, and some cities have regulated outdoors smoking areas. Cigarettes are no longer the same as in the past. The era of fashion trends was gone. Nowadays, smokers who smoke in public will only attract people's disgusting and disdainful eyes.

I've heard some people complained about this: smoking used to be fashionable, I followed it. At that time, there were cigarette advertisements and smokers everywhere. It's inconvenient to smoke anywhere now, but the old habits die hard.

The so-called fashion and masculinity are all Cigarette manufacturers' marketing tricks. They combine tobacco products with the image that young people aspire to: such as the Virginia Slims cigarettes combine smoking with a hot, young and beautiful female image; Marlboro cigarettes confuse smoking with masculinity; Mild Seven cigarettes cover product disputes with dynamic sports activities. When anti-smoking awareness has become the mainstream of the world, Cigarette manufacturers gradually change obvious advertisements into other forms of promotion, including paid advertisements such as radio, magazines, newspapers, outdoor billboards, mobile car bodies and various promotional activities, such as sponsoring arts and sports activities, investing in international racing competitions or well-known sports events.

But the fact is that smoking has nothing to do with the characteristics of cigarette advertisements (masculinity, hot body...), it's just bullshit. It's as ridiculous as the following advertisement, which says: I use this brand of cigarettes to protect my voice.

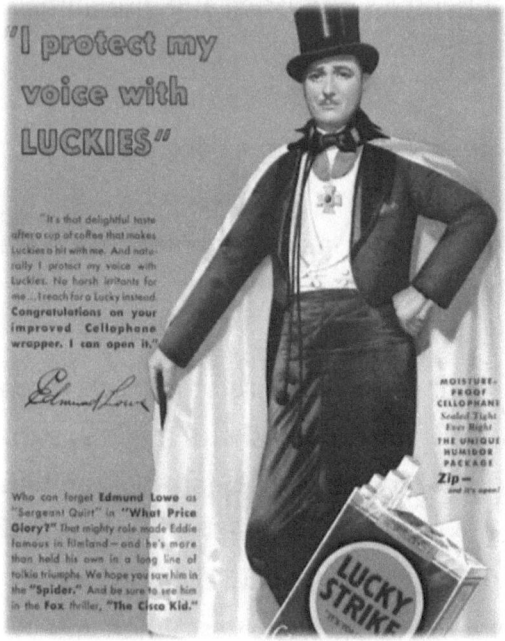

(In 1920s, a new wave in cigarette advertising: celebrity endorsements. Lucky Strike used this tactic extensively. The man in the poster was Edmund Lowe, an American actor, who died of lung cancer.)

You must know that smoking only increases your sputum and muddies your voice. But this advertisement claimed the cigarettes were able to maintain the voice. Wasn't it too exaggerating to deceive people like this?

This advertising poster has been almost a hundred years old. It is not difficult to see through the poster that the decrees on the management of cigarettes were so lax that cigarette manufacturers could make such a false advertising poster. Consumers of that era probably did not have enough information to distinguish the authenticity of advertising content. But from another angle, another few decades later from now, would it be an obvious deceptive trick when our descendants see the marketing methods of the current cigarette manufacturers.

What cigarette manufacturers are doing now is the same as they did 100 years ago. Those are:

◎ **In the past, they directly promoted their products and said that their products were good, but now they can't. Instead, they go to sponsorship activities to create an image that they are good, honest companies.**
◎ **Everyone is their potential customer. For those who don't smoke, they want you to try it. If they are already smokers, they want you to try their brand.**
◎ **They are constantly improving their product formulas, hoping to make people addicted faster, or making people more inseparable from their brand.**

Every brand of cigarette manufacturers is very clear about the positioning and segmentation of their brands in the market. There are almost no two brands of cigarette advertising appeals overlapping. I doubt that these different brands are actually the same company.

Operate the market with different brands to achieve higher market share.

For cigarette manufacturers, investing in advertising is very cost-effective. Whether you smoke or not, once you've crossed the threshold of smoking and become an addict, the rest will be handled by nicotine, which will help cigarette manufacturers get everything done and make smokers fall deeper and deeper, like the insect caught in a spider web.

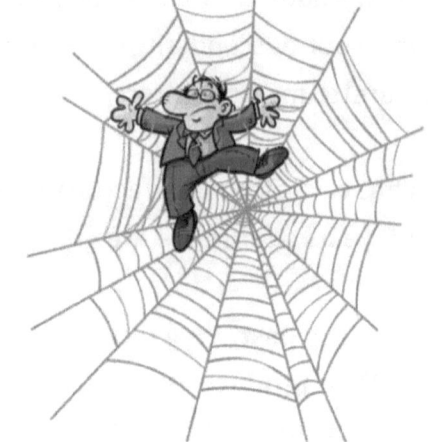

(Addiction is like spider web.)

(The reason quitting smoking is unsuccessful is that the previous smoking situation has always been remembered.)

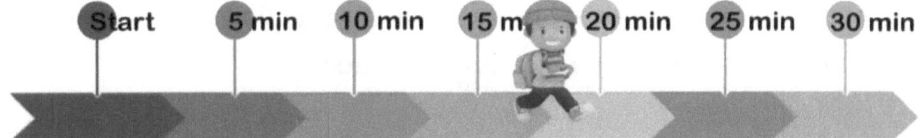

Reason 3: Cigarettes help to relax.

For a smoker, smoking is pleasant most of the time, right?

After waking up, eating, taking a dump, having sex, going to bed, talking about things... These are specific moments of a day; almost all of them are the time for smoking, and then you can proceed smoothly to the next stage.

But, do you know that the schedule of all this, which stage you need to smoke, how many cigarettes at least you need to smoke a day, is ingeniously arranged by the cigarette manufacturer. As long as you follow this schedule, you will feel happy, otherwise, you will begin to feel the call of cigarettes, gradually become the pull of cigarettes. Only after smoking a cigarette, you can be relieved.

Cigarette manufacturers know the time of nicotine metabolism in the body after smoking a cigarette. Every time you put out cigarettes, the concentration of nicotine in your body decreases over time, and so does the dopamine in your brain, and the brain that is accustomed to nicotine stimulation to produce dopamine will signal the demand for nicotine. If you don't give it to the brain, its reaction will become more and more intense, which is called addiction.

However, do you still remember, wasn't there anything that could make you satisfy and relax you before you addicted to smoking?

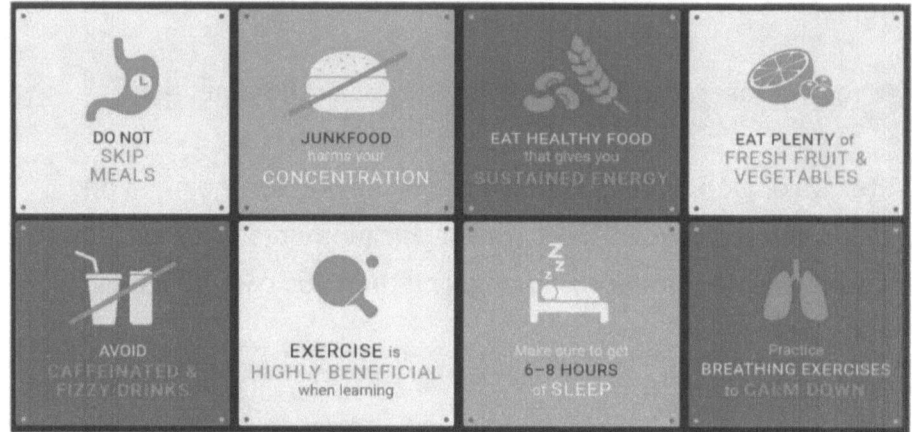

(These things can really help you relax.)

Of course, and a lot, right? But when you become addicted to cigarettes, you ignore things that are simple enough to make you soothe, relax, satisfy, and concentrate. No matter what you did, you have to smoke another cigarette to satisfy you. Otherwise, you will always feel that you are still missing something. This is the result of nicotine addiction, which reduces your sensitivity to other things and focuses only on smoking. We can find this phenomenon through experiments later.

Before your brain is addicted to nicotine, you could be satisfied with different things. It should be put this way: Whether you are satisfied or happy depends on you and the thing itself, not smoking. Just like many people like to smoke a cigarette after eating a meal, this made them feel satisfied, and then they thought that this is caused by the powerful effect of cigarettes. It is really a big mistake. This is because the interval between two cigarettes before and after the meal is long enough to reduce nicotine in the body to the level of demand, and the blood is concentrated in the stomach after meals. With the carbon monoxide produced by smoking which causes dizziness, so there will be an illusion of satisfaction and relaxation.

In fact, such satisfaction is more like self-abuse. This is just the same as after half-squatting for an hour, you are tired to death, then sitting down to rest, feeling relaxed. Whether you can get satisfaction from your meal depends on the delicacy of the food and the atmosphere during the meal. How can it be cigarettes?

We might as well do an experiment, which proves that the satisfaction of smoking after meals is entirely due to the demand for nicotine in the body, rather than the fact that cigarettes add to the delicacy of the food. Instead, people who are not addicted to cigarettes can really feel the satisfaction of food after meals.

The experimental contents are as follows:

- ◎ **Before eating, smoke a cigarette.**
- ◎ **Then continue to smoke while eating.**
- ◎ **The interval between each cigarette should not exceed five minutes to maintain the concentration of nicotine in the body.**
- ◎ **After eating, smoke another cigarette.**

After completing this experiment, you will find that the satisfaction of the original cigarette after the meal is gone. On the contrary, you will feel a little disgusting. The mouth is full of the tar smell of cigarettes, and you can't feel the original taste of the food.

During the day, everyone's mood, endocrine, and feelings will be somewhat ups and downs, sometimes excited, and sometimes depressed, but most of the time it is maintained in a neutral normal state, as shown in the chart below.

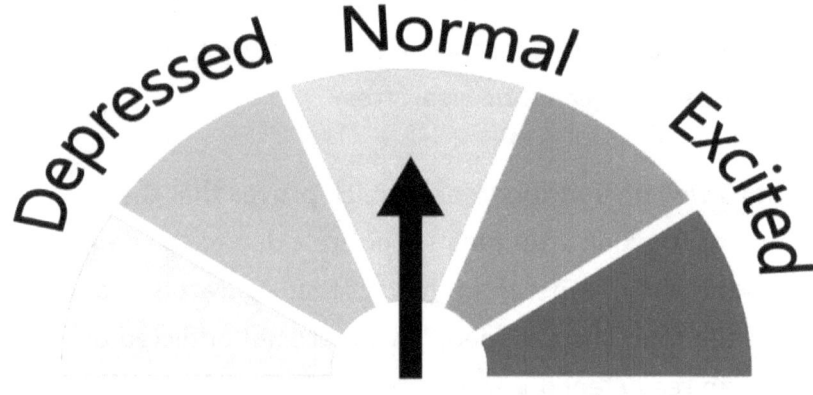

(Balanced state before addiction)

People who just started smoking, because the body has not adapted to the unexpected amount of nicotine, will feel dizzy, headache, nausea, palpitations... these uncomfortable feelings. At this time, nicotine makes the endocrine constant imbalance in the body, and the body has to adjust the amount of dopamine caused by nicotine. When the body gradually gets used to these uncomfortable reactions, the brain rebalances the original neutral constant state and shifts the neutral point toward the exciting end that affected by nicotine.

Once the new equilibrium is formed, it means that the brain has become addicted to nicotine. If you want to change the balance point, whether it is going to the higher level or the lower level, it will make the body suffer and uncomfortable again. Then, after a period of adaptation, a balance point will be generated.

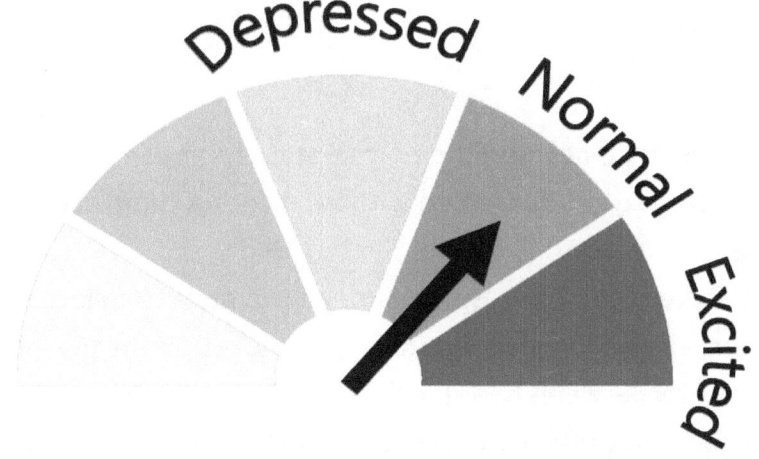

(Balanced state after addiction)

However, because of the new balance point (balanced state after addiction), it is caused by the stimulation of nicotine. Once the content of nicotine in the body decreases, it is easy to feel anxiety, stress, disturbance, irritability, etc. Even if it only returns to the endocrine level before the addiction, but because of the stimulation of nicotine, smokers will be depressed due to the stimulation of nicotine... withdrawal symptoms.

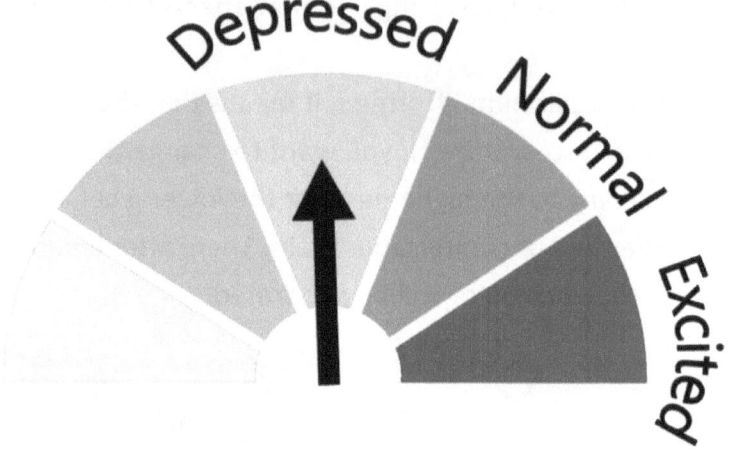

(After addicted, because the normal state has been lifted up, so it's easy to get depressed without nicotine stimulation.)

When depression occurs, smokers need to smoke to relieve the situation. The fewer years of smoking a smoker are, or the longer the time interval between two smoking sessions, or when the cigarette is lit, the first few puffs of the cigarette inhaled are the most prone to excitement.

However, as the age of smoking increases and the time of smoking becomes denser, the more difficult it is for nicotine to satisfy the brain, the harder it is to reach a state of excitement, but it is more likely to fall into a low mood because of insufficient smoking. As to the smoker with longer years of smoking, because smoking can only make the dopamine level of the brain return to the low level of the normal state, so he must change to smoke the heavier cigarettes or increase the number of cigarettes, and become a chain smoker.

(When a craving comes, you can still insist on quitting smoking, it is the real quit smoking... You have quit smoking for 20 minutes, stick to it)

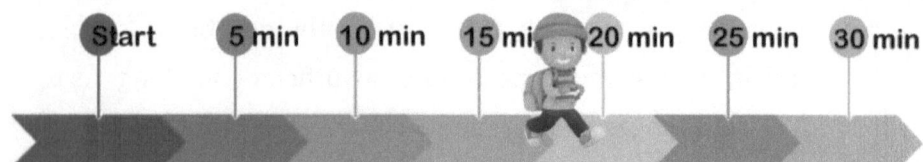

Start   5 min   10 min   15 min   20 min   25 min   30 min

Reason 4: Smoking makes the stool smoother.

Some people who quit smoking say, "I used to have a good bowel movement. Why do I start constipation after quitting smoking?" or "I can't defecate without smoking" Are these excuses for not to quit smoking?

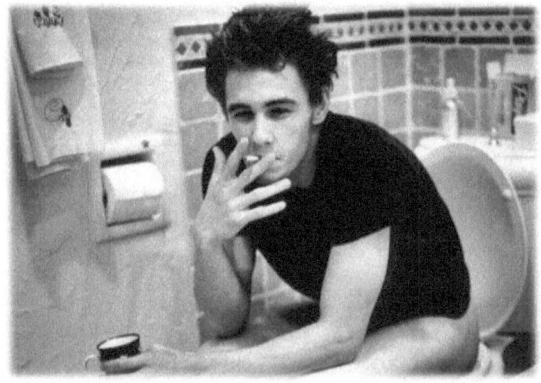

(Smoking can solve defecating problem? Why not try enema? If using enema is ridiculous, so does smoking.)

It's true. It happened to me. It is theoretically inferred that nicotine and tar from cigarettes stimulate gastrointestinal peristalsis when you start smoking and make you feel want to defecate. For some people with constipation, smoking can kill two birds with one stone, which can relieve addiction and defecate.

But if you continue to smoke for a reason like this, isn't it the same as drinking the sea water to quench thirst when drifting on the sea. Moreover, when the body gets used to the concentration of nicotine, it will be paralyzed, and then there will be constipation problems again. Sometimes, smoking too much may cause mild nicotine poisoning nausea, vomiting or diarrhea.

Besides anxiety, irritability, depression and other emotional withdrawal symptoms when quitting smoking, there will also be some physical discomfort, which is a great challenge to willpower. The following are some common physical discomforts during smoking cessation:

Thirst: Thirsty often accompanies smoking cessation. Drinking plenty of water helps to metabolize nicotine in the body.

Sleep interruption: Wake up halfway through the night, and then you can't sleep. This is one of the most painful withdrawal symptoms, and it is very common.

Drowsiness: Smokers may have a greater sense of relaxation without the chemical refreshing effect of nicotine. Some people feel that they can fall asleep at any time. Taking a nap after a meal and extending the night's sleep time may help to overcome this situation.

Insomnia at night: Some people find it difficult to fall asleep at night after stopping smoking. You can use your time to get up, read or take a walk, and don't lie in bed to force yourself to fall asleep. Do not drink caffeinated beverages such as tea, coffee, cocoa, cola, etc. before going to bed.

Cough: After years of smoking, the lungs produce a lot of self-protecting mucus. After starting to quit smoking, the mucus will become thinner and looser, expelled from the respiratory tract, and the cilia will start to re-sport, so people who quit smoking will usually experience coughing for a while.

Headache: Some people have headaches, sometimes lasting for a day. The reason is that the microvessels of the brain are no longer contracted, which were stimulated by nicotine, and that makes the blood flow well and the nerves are more sensitive. You can drink some coffee, and caffeine helps to relieve headaches.

Hunger: The body's ability to absorb food has improved. Almost all smokers have a better appetite after quitting smoking. In order to avoid gaining weight, you can do some physical exercise and eat low-sugar and low-calorie foods.

Night sweats: Some smokers who were heavily addicted to cigarettes will experience night sweats while sleeping. It was found that the lack of nicotine causes dysautonomia, the disorder of the self-discipline nervous system. Exercise can alleviate this situation.

Tremor: The hand and fingers tremble slightly, also because the endocrine is affected by the lack of nicotine, which makes the autonomic nervous system disorder (dysautonomia).

Mouth sores: a few people who quit smoking may have oral irritation. Gingival blistering, aphthous ulcers, or inflammation are caused by the change of chemical substances in the body. Vitamin deficiency may cause it. Strengthening nutrition and vitamin B and C supplementation can ease symptoms.

Inattention: After the concentration of carbon monoxide in the body decreases, it may affect the sense of space and distance during smoking cessation, and the results are the feeling of floating and difficulty in concentration, but the situation should not be too serious.

Hand and foot itching or scalp soreness: This is caused by the tightening of capillaries without nicotine stimulation and the improvement of the circulatory system, which rarely lasts long.

Many smokers pay little attention to their health, especially in diet. This may be because smokers believe that smoking itself is the greatest harm to the body. Other things, such as diet, work and rest, exercise, etc., even if you pay little attention, it won't have much effect on your health. Of course, such an idea is wrong.

The good news is that if constipation is only caused by smoking cessation, not any other psychological factors, after adding food fiber, taking more fresh fruits and vegetables, and drinking more water, it can be quickly eliminated, and it is unnecessary to hinder smoking cessation because of such things at all, and it is also unnecessary to use drugs or enema to make defecation smooth.

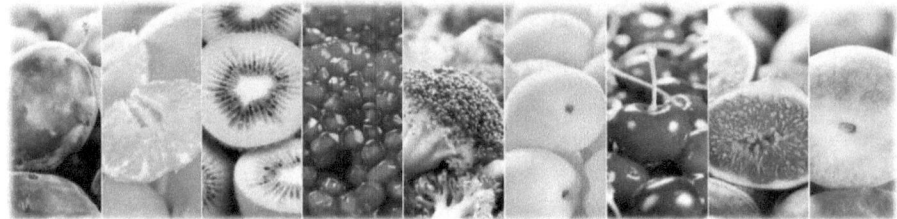

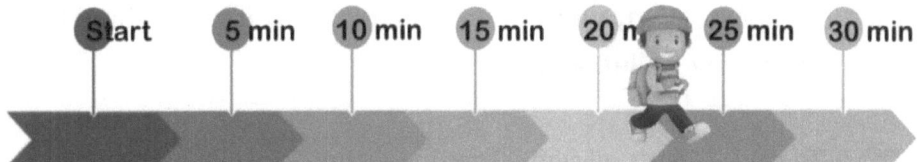

Start   5 min   10 min   15 min   20 m   25 min   30 min

Reason 5: There is no sense of security without carrying cigarettes on.

On a cool fall evening, my wife and I were walking in the street.

The rush hour had passed, there were not too many vehicles on the street, nor passers-by in a hurry. Most of the pedestrians were residents of this neighborhood. When people meet, they nodded their heads cordially.

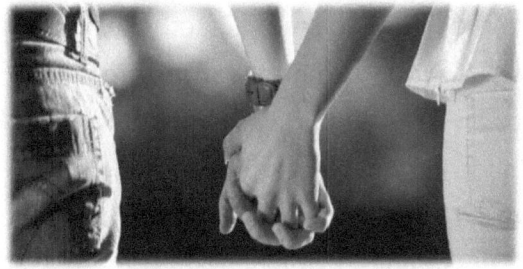

(Don't let cigarettes come between your hands.)

My wife and I passed a supermarket. This supermarket was sure to pass every time we walk. The wife proposed to go shopping and buy some fruit.

I hadn't quit smoking yet. I was planning smoking outside the supermarket while my wife went shopping for fruit inside. But I found I didn't bring my wallet with me.

The wife said, "That's all right. Then don't buy it. We'll buy it tomorrow. Let's go on walking."

Then I found that I had forgotten to bring cigarettes. I didn't care about going out without my wallet, nor did I want to smoke. But when I found the cigarettes were not on me and I couldn't buy them, I became panicked. I couldn't go on walking at all and became keen to smoke.

Just at this moment, I met my neighbor Jackson, who was also a smoker. He just bought something from the supermarket. I knew he must have cigarettes, so I asked him for one.

Afterward, I thought back, why did I have to smoke? Actually, I didn't know what happened to myself. Although I didn't want to smoke, I knew that I had not smoked for an hour, and it was almost time for the craving. At this time, I didn't bring the cigarette with me. This situation made me feel flustered, I had to find a cigarette to smoke first, to avoid the suffering of the craving of smoking.

We didn't go on walking that night but walked home quickly. The good mood of walking with my wife was ruined by the lack of cigarettes.

Looking back now, I feel that I was really ridiculous. It seemed I became a person without a soul, like a puppet of cigarettes. I have to be obedient to the cigarette and let it left its mercy on me.

This situation is not confined to going out, but also at home. Basically, whether at home, in my office, in my car... anywhere, as long as I might stay for over 30 minutes, there would be plenty of cigarettes.

To tell you the truth, I'm not sure whether I bought so many cigarettes to store in order to make it convenient for me to have cigarettes anytime I want to smoke, or did the manufacturer of cigarettes lay a grub on me?

Until my wife said to me one day, "Hubby, why do you smoke more and more cigarettes?" I realized that I had inadvertently stored a lot of cigarettes.

For a non-smoker, it's better to pick up a coin on the street than a pack of cigarettes. But for smokers, cigarettes are valuable. How valuable are they? If a pack of cigarettes and the money equivalent to the cigarettes were both put on the table to let the smoker choose, the smoker will choose cigarettes instead of money without hesitation, because choosing cigarettes means he can smoke immediately, but choosing money means he has to spend more time to buy them.

For a smoker, it is unlikely to quit smoking with a lot of cigarettes in stock. Because smokers feel that if they quit smoking, what about the cigarettes that have not been smoked? He believes that he should wait until he has finished smoking all the cigarettes he stocked, so he will not waste any cigarettes. But the problem is that smokers couldn't even allow no cigarettes around them, and as long as the cigarettes are below a certain safe amount, he will buy them again.

This is the insecurity caused by tobacco addiction, so the smoker will continue to buy cigarettes and smoke to satisfy his insecurity.

Smoking addiction is like a devil hidden in your body, constantly driving you to buy and smoke to fill it. You are afraid that if you don't have a cigarette, you will be occupied by the addiction of cigarettes and feel uncomfortable. Because of this, it is so difficult to quit

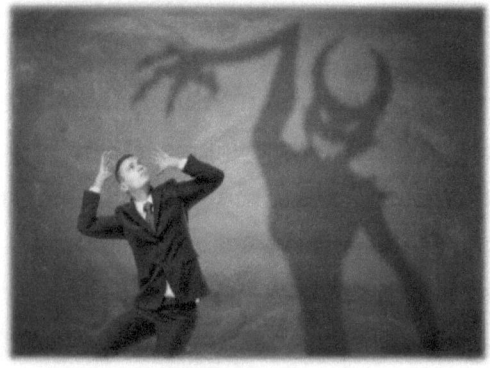 smoking.

In fact, when you first try to smoke, you have to work hard to "learn." When you smoke the first cigarette, it will definitely cause a cough. If you smoke too much for the first

(Addictions are demons.)

time, you will also experience dizziness, nausea, and other reactions. That's how our bodies express, "You've eaten the toxin into your body! Stop it! What does it mean? Attitudes towards this reaction often determine whether we will be addicted to tobacco.

Many people think only weak-willed people will become addicted to tobacco, which is actually wrong. Weak-minded people are usually lucky because they can't stand for the feeling of smoking the first cigarette, and their lungs can't tolerate the suffocation caused by inhaling cigarette-burning gases, so they won't smoke for a lifetime. Or they can't accept the pain of smoking psychologically, so they won't try again.

For those who are addicted to cigarettes, that it takes a lot of effort to "learn" smoking is one of the greatest tragedies. Many smokers think they really like the smell of smoke, which is actually an illusion. When we "learn" smoking, we are actually forcing the body to adapt to the bad smell of smoke. Heroin addicts also believe that they like the feeling of heroin injection, but the fact is that heroin withdrawal symptoms are more painful, they like pain relief when injecting heroin.

If a smoker believes that he only smokes because he likes the taste of cigarettes, you can ask him, "If you don't have the brand of cigarettes you usually smoke, only the brand you don't like, will you take it?" Of course he will. Moreover, neither cold, flu, sore throat, tracheitis nor emphysema can prevent smokers from lighting up a cigarette.

So the best way to deal with the insecurities of smoking addiction is to ignore it, it will naturally disappear. When the body lacks nicotine and

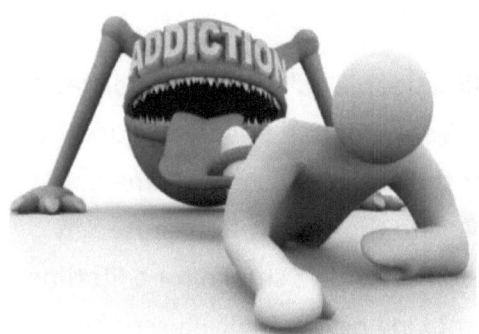

feels uneasy, it means that the demon in your body is uncomfortable and protesting, hoping you would feed it; but if you keep feeding it, it will only ask for more, and make your smoke more.

(Defeat the addiction or be eaten.)

Part 1 QUIZ

1. How many times have you tried to quit smoking?
   a. None   +1
   b. Once   +2
   c. Twice   +3
   d. Three times   +4
   e. Over Three times   +5

2. What's the reason you've been smoking all these years?
   a. The cigarette tastes great   +3
   b. Increased self-confidence   +3
   c. Relax   +3
   d. Social   +3
   e. Cigarette addiction   +1
   f. All of the above   +5

3. If time goes back, would you still want to become addicted to tobacco?
   a. Yes   +5
   b. No   +1
   c. I am not sure   +3

4. What makes you want to quit smoking?
   a. Healthy   +3

b. Family   +3

c. Money   +3

d. Tired of smoking   +1

Before moving to next stage, please check your points at the end of each options and add them up first. If the points are below "8", welcome to the next page. Otherwise, I strongly recommend you start over and re-establish your perception of cigarettes.

5. Please write down your expectations for quitting smoking in a few simple words:

6. Who is the biggest beneficiary behind cigarettes?
   a. Tobacco farmers
   b. Cigarette manufacturers
   c. The government

• Part 2 •

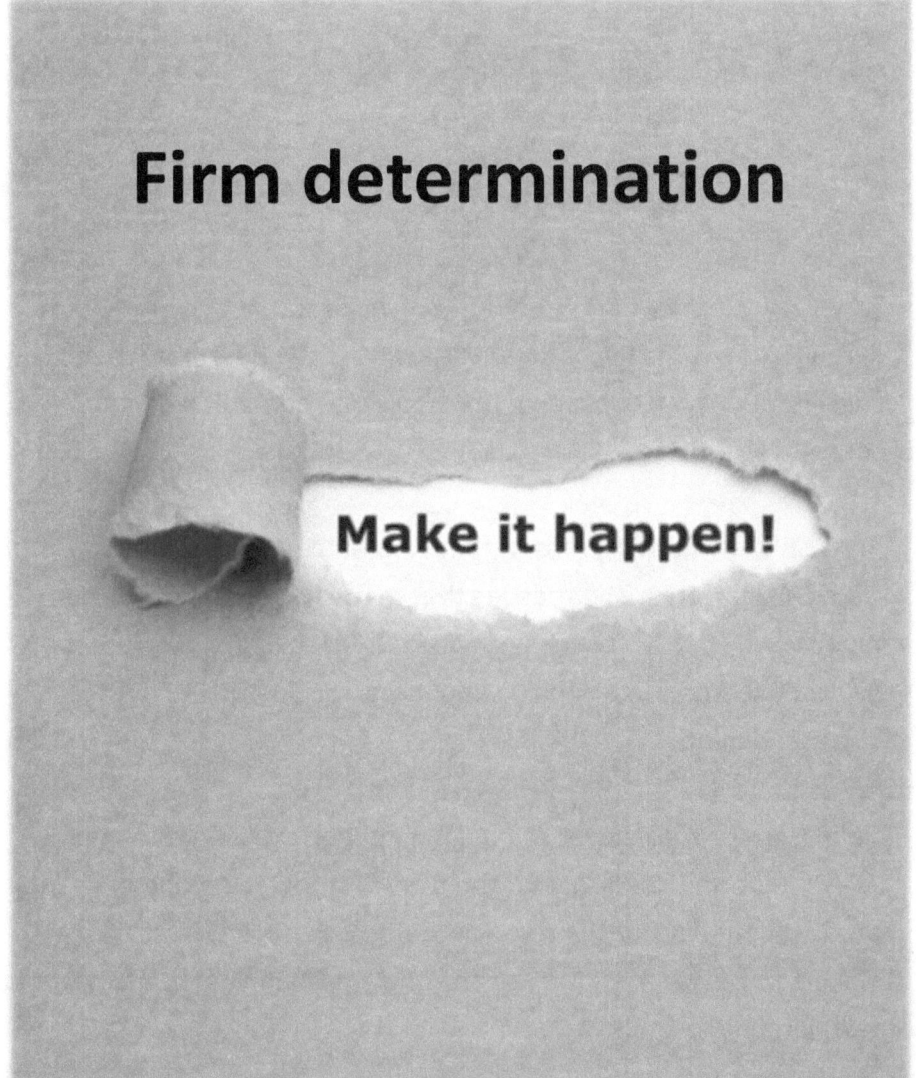

Firm determination

Make it happen!

(A person who has experienced smoking cessation knows the suffering before the disappearance of the craving, so he does not want to fall into the trap again.)

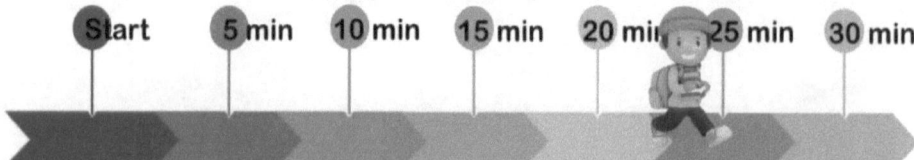

Strengthen your beliefs

If you are spontaneous and don't want to smoke anymore, but don't know which way to quit smoking is the best way, then congratulations, after reading this book, you can quit smoking successfully.

There isn't any quitting reason that can match your fundamental dislike of cigarettes. The reasons that made you smoke, whether influenced by peers, for social occasions, masculinity, depression, or any other reason, have long disappeared, leaving only cigarette addiction behind.

The reason for smoking at the beginning, perhaps in today's view, is so ridiculous and childish, and the former smoking companions may have lost contact, but the remaining smoking addiction, driving smokers to buy and smoke day after day, probably was unexpected at the beginning of smoking.

If people can't be autonomous but manipulated by others, it is like a puppet. But the same thing happens to other creatures. "Zombie ants" is an example. There is a unique fungus in nature that controls

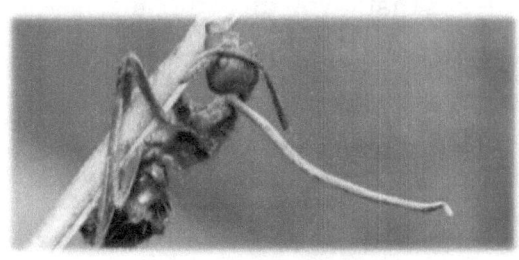

the behavior of ants by releasing chemicals, so the ants help the fungus find a suitable growth environment, manipulated by the fungi, and finally killed by the fungi.

(A dead zombie ant)

Ants controlled by fungi will no longer have their own behaviors and lives, and the final stages of their lives are also the most painful and horrible. In the last few hours of life, "Zombie Ants" will crawl below the leaves where they are, and bite the central veins of the leaves with their jaws, trapping themselves on the leaves. At the same time, the parasitic fungus can also attach to the leaves, and the leaves become the ants' graveyards.

Looking at the picture, an ant hangs on the branch and bites the twig tightly. You might think this is a normal ant. In fact, it is a zombie ant that can't control itself!

Fortunately, although we are controlled by cigarettes, we can still have our own consciousness and choose to give up smoking, not as ants, once infected, they will be enslaved by fungi for life and eventually be killed.

If you quit smoking because of your doctor's warning and for health reasons, congratulations. This means that if you quit smoking, it will be very helpful for your recovery, so the doctor asked you to quit smoking. On the contrary, for a patient who is terminally ill and can't be cured, the doctor wouldn't ask him to quit smoking. He would say, "Do whatever you want."

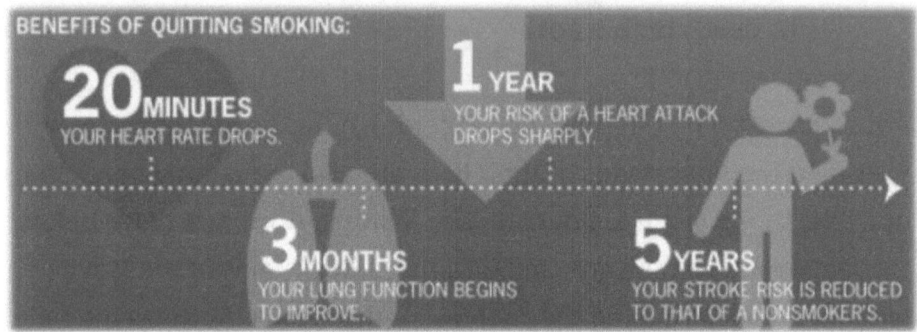

(Benefits of quitting smoking)

Once you stop smoking, it almost instantly helps your body. Quitting smoking can help the heart rate and blood pressure gradually return to normal, improve lung function, reduce the occurrence of heart disease, stroke, nasopharyngeal, laryngeal cancer, and other diseases.

From the first day of smoking cessation, the body's carbon monoxide, nicotine, and other substances will be slowly excreted by the body. After successful smoking cessation, the health of the body's major organs will be restored to the same level as non-smokers, and the skin can also be improved.

When smoking, the concentration of carbon monoxide in the body increases, inhibiting the oxygen-carrying capacity of red blood cells in the body and makes the body in a situation where the oxygen content and oxygen saturation of the blood are reduced, and the blood circulation of the body is blocked. After stopping smoking, the blood circulation of the whole body is improved, these symptoms are alleviated, and the blood circulation of the body can return to normal.

Many people mistakenly believe that smoking is a way to relieve stress. That's because of nicotine addiction, giving people a temporary psychological satisfaction through smoking. This satisfaction is temporary, and it can't really improving mental stress. After quitting smoking, the improvement of respiratory system function can help the body to inhale more oxygen, which can help the body to get more oxygen supplement and relieve stress.

Quitting smoking for the sake of family members is something that many parents who are about to have newborn babies will do. But I don't know if it's because some people are forced to give up smoking because of this reason, the success rate is lower, and the probability of smoking again in the future is higher. But it's always good to try to quit smoking. If you can skip one cigarette today, you may skip a pack of cigarettes tomorrow.

I'm sure you've heard a lot about the dangers of second-hand smoking. But second-hand smoke is not only smoke from smokers, but also smoke directly released into the air during the burning process of cigarettes, which is not inhaled by smokers.

In addition, pregnant women can pass the chemicals and nicotine in the cigarettes to the fetus through the blood, resulting in low birth weight and a higher risk of sudden infant death. Even if a woman does not smoke, as long as someone in the family is a smoker, harmful substances will be passed on to the fetus because of inhalation of second-hand smoke.

Secondhand smoke has negative effects on the health of pregnant women, fetuses and their various growth stages, which is recognized by the medical research. Pregnant women inhaling second-hand smoke will pass harmful substances to the fetus through the placenta. Fetuses in pregnant women have a much higher absorption of carbon monoxide than adults. The developing organs of the fetus will face the hypoxia state of oxygen deficiency, and the hypoxia during childbirth, the emergency laparotomy is needed. During pregnancy, there may be acute or chronic symptoms such as abortion, premature birth, stillbirth, low fetal weight, thoracic infection, sudden death of newborns, fetal malformations, and fetal pulmonary insufficiency. Some diseases cannot be cured and can last a lifetime or threaten the fetus life.

So, if you quit smoking for your family or the next generation, maybe

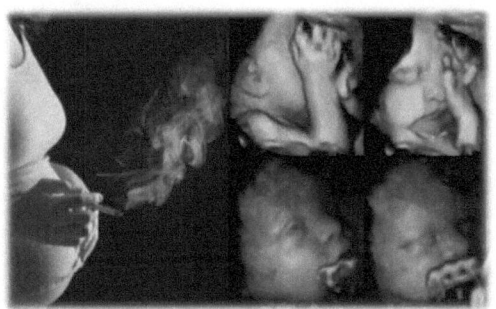

your quitting process will be more laborious than others, but your family will deeply feel your efforts and thank you for being a good husband (wife) or a good father (mother).

(Smoking chokes the fetus.)

Quitting smoking in order to save money. It is not because you can't afford to smoke, but you are unwilling to be exploited again

The cost of a pack of cigarette ingredients is extremely low, and many of the costs are spent on advertising and marketing. But why are cigarettes so expensive? How expensive is it?

From the chart on next page you can see the price of Marlboro worldwide. In Pakistan, Vietnam, the darkest green country, it sold for $1, but in the deepest red Australia, the same pack of cigarettes cost $20.66.

The biggest difference is the amount of tax collected by the government. In the United States, although Marlboro is also the same, the price in each state is different. Most states or cities are around $7, but in New York City, a pack costs $13.

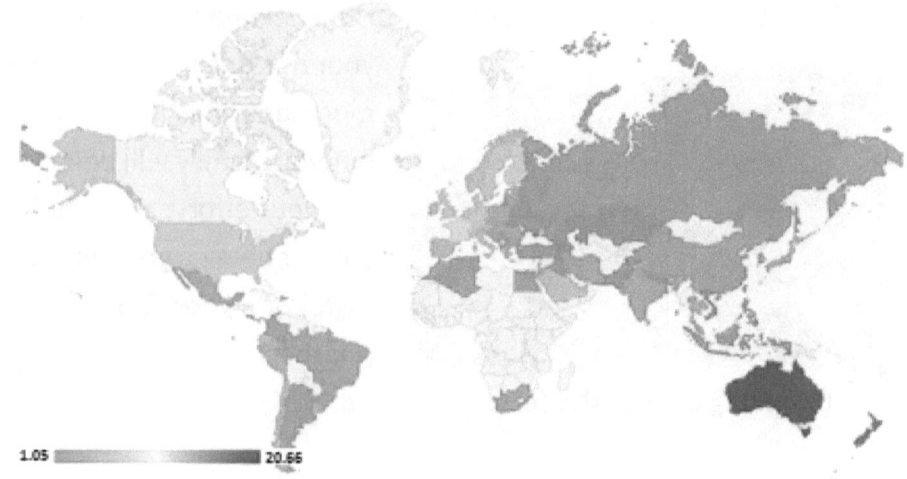

1.05 — 20.66

(Marlboro 20 Pack, currency: USD)

Most governments draw 75% of the price of cigarettes as taxes, but some cities or countries are higher. Even in the cheapest countries, the government still draws taxes, but it only draws fewer taxes on cigarettes. But no matter in which country or city, these cigarettes are exactly the same, but the difference in price shows how low the cost of the cigarette itself is.

Basically, most governments regard cigarettes as "unwelcome goods." Not only do they impose heavy taxes on commodities, but they also impose heavy taxes on local manufacturers with factories and employees.

Please don't think this tax is unreasonable. Before I quit smoking, I thought the tax was unreasonable, too. But now I don't know how much the tax for a pack of cigarettes is and I don't care, because it's not my business.

Before I quit smoking, what I felt unfair is: Cigarettes are essential for people's livelihood. Why should we pay heavy taxes? If the government does not welcome cigarettes, then simply ban people from smoking. I even called the IRS, the government's tax department, and asked them why cigarettes were taxed heavily. The answer is: "Cigarettes are not essential for people's livelihood, but products that are harmful to health. Of course, you have to pay a heavy tax. If you think it is too expensive, you may choose not to buy it, don't smoke it, and no one forces you to buy it."

Smokers, please always remember: no one forces you to smoke, you learned how to smoke yourselves, you chose to be addicted; No one forces you to continue smoking. You want to buy and smoke cigarettes voluntarily. Since everything is voluntary, you can only be willing to be taxed heavily.

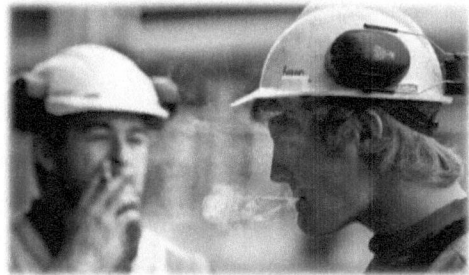

(Many workers think that smoking is a kind of leisure when taking a break.)

Although many smokers are blue-collar workers and lower income laborers, smoking is a big expense for them, but in the government's view, smokers are not a vulnerable group. Those who can afford to buy cigarettes represent those who can afford to buy luxury goods.

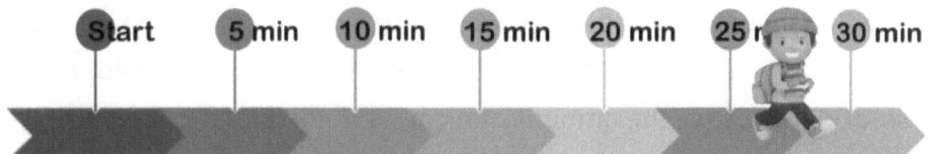

(Since you decided to quit smoking, it is already better than others)

Start · 5 min · 10 min · 15 min · 20 min · 25 min · 30 min

Never use any substitutes to help you

quit smoking

A gain, don't quit smoking with any substitutes, really. The most important step in quitting smoking is to make up your mind. So far, you have done a good job.

You haven't smoked for nearly 30 minutes. Just continue your thoughts for the past 30 minutes and keep doing so. As for how to relieve the discomfort feeling when withdrawal symptoms occur will be explained in the later article.

Using other things to help you quit smoking will only make you fall into another trap; especially nicotine products like nicotine patches, nicotine chewable tablets, nicotine inhalers, these things will only make your time to quit smoking even longer and may lead to a failure to quit smoking.

The principle of nicotine products is to add nicotine ingredients to chewing tablets, patches, or filters. When smokers use these products, nicotine ingredients are absorbed through the mouth and skin, into the blood, and recycled to the brain. People who are addicted to smoking, because the amount of nicotine in the blood is insufficient, the brain will be stimulated and give smoking instructions to supplement the amount of nicotine in the body.

Nicotine products, by supplementing nicotine in the blood, keeping the concentration of nicotine in blood not to drop too fast, so the smokers won't have to bear the depression symptoms during withdrawal.

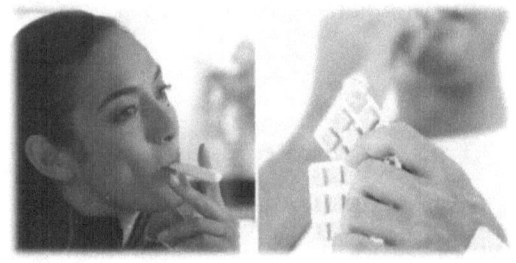

(Nicotine products are not made for quitting smoking, but to replace cigarettes.)

But when we quit smoking, the main purpose is to quit the addiction caused by nicotine, so stop smoking and make the brain get no supply of nicotine. Finally, the brain gave up the need for nicotine because of disappointment and achieved the purpose of quitting smoking. If we continue to provide nicotine in other ways at this time, the brain will expect to get nicotine continuously, because of the new source.

The reason why smokers who use nicotine products to quit smoking would eventually fail is that it is more troublesome to use nicotine products than smoking. The smokers will think: "Since I'm absorbing nicotine, I'd rather smoke less than using patches." And turn back to smoking again. Otherwise, smokers feel that nicotine products can't give them the same excitement as cigarettes. In addition to using nicotine products, they also smoke a few more cigarettes. The result is, of course, the opposite.

As we discussed earlier, quitting smoking is like breaking up in a lovelorn relationship. Let's assume a very bad situation, you might as well think about it: if your girlfriend is unfaithful to you, dating someone else. You noticed the situation and she regrets what she did, wants to break up with that person. Which kind of breakup do you think is the real breakup? Never see each other nor any longer contact, or occasionally meet, call, and send a message? Similarly, if someone tells you that he is using a nicotine patch to quit smoking, would you think he quit smoking successfully? Of course not! Not only that, it takes a long time to use nicotine products to quit smoking. Usually, a course of treatment is three months to half a year; but the way you quit smoking now, in about three weeks, you can feel walking out of the haze of smoking addiction.

As for e-cigarettes, it is not a product that helps you quit smoking, but a substitute for cigarettes for people who don't want to quit. If you don't want to quit smoking, you want to smoke conveniently anytime and anywhere besides the usual smoking, then use e-cigarettes. It's a big mistake that many people wrongly think e-cigarettes are healthier because they don't have a choking smell. Every e-cigarette you smoke is chemically synthesized. It's totally unregistered, unregulated, and the factory is not qualified either. Instead of smoking e-cigarettes, you might as well continue smoking cigarettes.

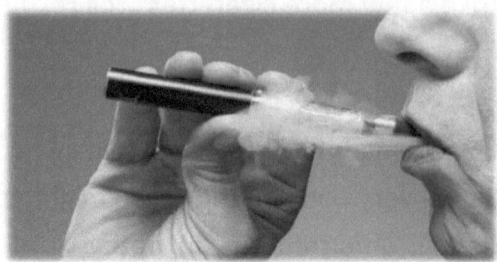

(You never know what e-cigarettes are made of.)

Some people switch to chewing gum and candy. It's also a terrible way to replace smoking. Don't think it doesn't matter that changing to something else, which is not addictive. On the surface, it may not be as bad as smoking, but over time, it will become a habit and dependence, and it is also prone to obesity. It's just like when you're lovelorn, to make yourself feel better, you go to find somebody to replace the one you previously loved. After a while, you get out of the sadness of the lovelorn, but you realized the one of replacement around you is not suitable, but you've got used to her. If you break up again, you'll have pain again.

Another thing many people don't know is that carbohydrates, including sugar, are harder to quit than cigarettes. The reason is that they are all made into various products, appear around our lives, too easy to get, almost cannot avoid this kind of food, it is easy to eat too much unconsciously, resulting in overweight. And when you want to quit them, they are constantly appearing in front of you, even you have to eat them, because they are stapled foods, but cannot eat too much, it is really a difficult and painful thing.

So, if you are not addicted to and dependent on carbohydrates, sugar, don't let yourself eat more and more sugar unconsciously, and eventually become a habit. Otherwise, it will be a very headache and trouble. Sugar-containing foods are like the bees whose honeycomb had been stabbed, chasing you around and you can't get rid of them.

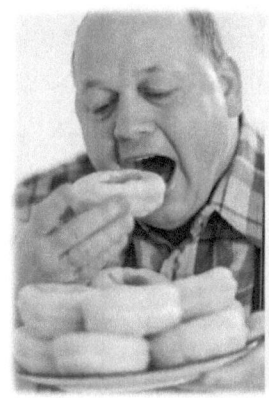 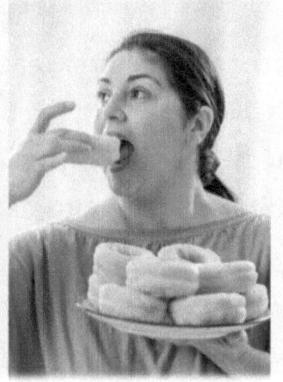 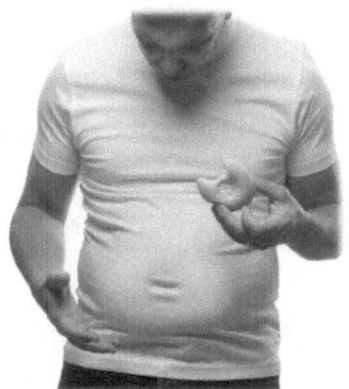

(Carbohydrates are harder to quit than cigarettes.)

(Congratulations, you've successfully passed the first 30 minutes without smoking.)

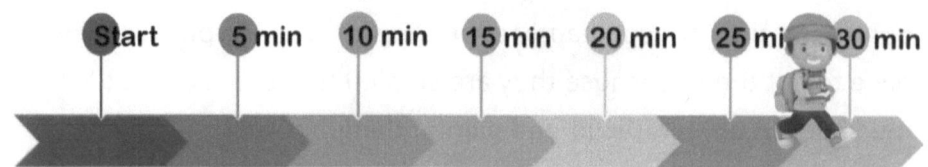

N. O. P. E, Not One Puff Ever.

One of the difficulties that many people face when they quit smoking is that they are waiting for the elimination of cravings.

If your goal is to run a marathon, then after reaching the end, you can tell yourself that you have achieved your goal. But when smokers quit smoking, they told themselves: "If I can stop smoking, after a long enough time, the craving will disappear naturally."

How long is "long enough"? You have no way to judge, you can only wait patiently, hoping that something can be used as a sign to let you know that quitting smoking has really succeeded. Many people would think that after quitting smoking successfully, they would return to non-addiction status, like they have never been addicted before, become non-smokers, or feel rejected and disgusted when they smoke.

So, some people will give themselves an excuse to take a PUFF to see if they are addicted. But as long as there is such an idea, it means that addiction still exists in the heart.

In fact, quitting smoking is successful at the moment you put out your last cigarette, but if you take a puff and try to find out if you still have cravings, what you are waiting for is just the moment when you fail to quit smoking > > > > the moment when you give in to yourself, because once you smoke again, you will fall into the circle of expecting the next cigarette. And for a person who doesn't smoke or who really quits smoking, it's not something that he wants to try.

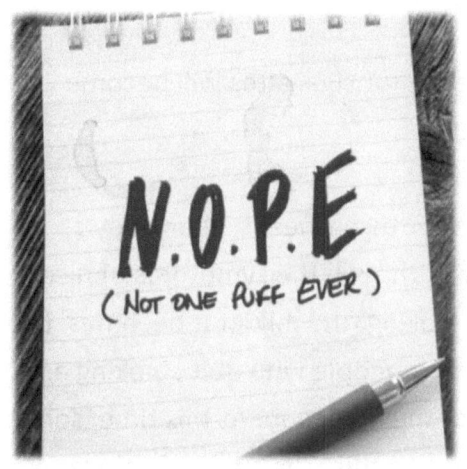

(N.O.P.E is very important.)

The psychological pain of smokers when they quit smoking is the result of hesitation and suspicion. Although there is no physical pain, psychological pain is also difficult to bear. You should have totally forgotten about smoking, but your consciousness is entangled.

This pain can last for a few days or even weeks. Your mind is full of such thoughts:

"How long will the cigarette craving last?"

"Can I still find happiness?"

"Would I like to get up every morning?"

"Can I still enjoy the time after dinner?"

"How can I relieve stress in the future?"

"How do I deal with social occasions?"

When you think that way, your desire for cigarettes will become stronger and stronger.

In fact, as long as you don't smoke for three weeks, your body's hunger for nicotine will disappear. Although the symptoms of nicotine withdrawal, the longer you stop smoking, the milder it becomes. But when the symptoms disappear, many people who quit smoking are still aware that they have got rid of the addiction. At this time, some people will light up a cigarette to prove this. The smell of smoke makes them feel bad, and it seems that addiction has disappeared. However, as a result, they ingested new nicotine, and after the cigarettes were extinguished, the withdrawal symptoms reappeared. They will think subconsciously: "I have to get another one." They had already got rid of the cravings, but they became re-addicted again.

They don't immediately light up a second cigarette, because they still have the mentality of "I can't repeat the same mistake", so they will wait for a while, after a few hours, a few days, a few weeks, until they feel safe. They will think, "It seems that I am really getting rid of the addiction, so it doesn't matter if I smoke one more now." But they did not know that they were slipping bit by bit into the trap they had already broken away.

Remember, you have started to quit smoking, and it has been half an hour since you just finished the last cigarette. During this half hour, you are pretty sure you want to quit smoking. You just have to concentrate on quitting smoking and keep your current non-smoking state. As for the case of cravings, ask yourself:

What is the reason I decided to quit smoking?
What are the benefits of smoking?
Do I really like smoking?

If the time without smoking is difficult, it is even more important to remember the time you spent, because those times are hard to accumulate. But just one puff, it will destroy the accumulated time, and everything has to start from scratch.

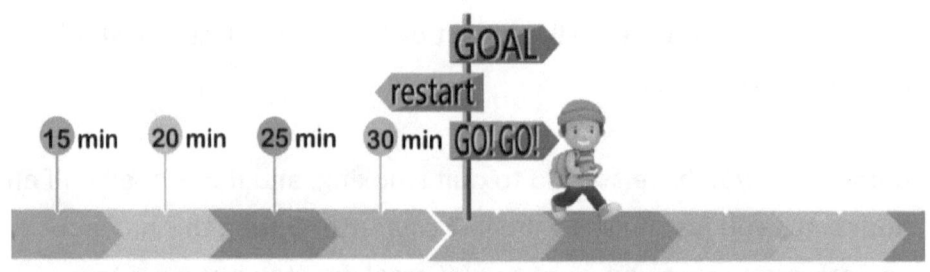

(It takes only five seconds for a puff, and the results of quitting are ruined.)

Eliminate Cravings Breathing Method

This is a breathing method. It takes 3 to 5 minutes to make smokers quickly eliminate the physiological discomfort caused by smoking addiction, increase the body's oxygen content, and improve the utilization rate of oxygen.

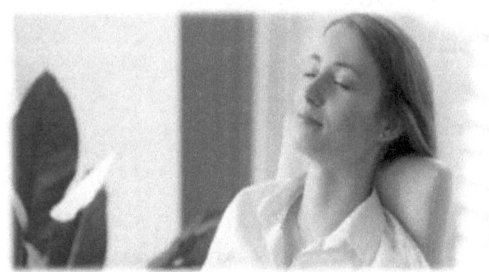

(Concentrate on breathing.)

When you are doing this breathing method, please fully concentrate on breathing, so the breathing method can play a major role.

You can always smoke at any time. Just like you used to, you can smoke whenever you want to. You haven't missed any chance, but you just don't want to do it.

Be sure to put away all the distractions thoughts in your head, concentrate on doing it, and do it slowly. Don't do Eliminate Cravings Breathing Method while still thinking about smoking. You can tell yourself this way: I am now focusing on Eliminate Cravings Breathing Method. If I finish it, I still feel that it is not working, I can't bear the cravings, and it's not too late to smoke.

Remember, you can smoke at any time, no one or anything will restrict you. The reason why you don't smoke again is that you are tough and you can endure the withdrawal symptoms of your body when you are not smoking, and you cherish the accumulated smoking cessation hours.

After you learned the breathing method, whenever you have a craving, use this method to breathe, and you can quickly defeat the craving.

◎ **There is no limit to the posture of the body, whether standing, sitting or lying.**
◎ **Prepare a stopwatch.**
◎ **Take 10 deep breaths, breathe evenly, empty your mind and concentrate on breathing.**
◎ **After the last inhalation, hold your breath and start timing.**
◎ **Stick to your limits as far as possible. Through practice, you can**

hold your breath longer and longer.

◎ After resuming breathing, take deep breaths until you feel relief.

◎ Keep a record of each time you hold the breath. In addition to slowly breaking through your own record, you can also observe the frequency of your cravings.

Eliminate Cravings Breathing			
Date	MM / DD	/	/
Time	00 : 00 Sec	: Sec	: Sec
	: Sec	: Sec	: Sec
	: Sec	: Sec	: Sec
	: Sec	: Sec	: Sec
	: Sec	: Sec	: Sec

(Put down your record in the table.)

Eliminate Cravings Breathing Method is designed for people who want to quit smoking, to eliminate cigarette cravings; if a person who has not made up his mind and does not want to quit smoking, and hopes to eliminate the cravings through Eliminate Cravings Breathing Method, then, even the addiction in the body has been eliminated, but the craving in the heart will be repeated.

In addition to helping to quit smoking, Eliminate Cravings Breathing Method can also increase lung capacity, blood oxygenation, and reduce carbon monoxide concentration in the body. Even after quitting smoking, you still can practice twice a day early and evening to calm your body and mind.

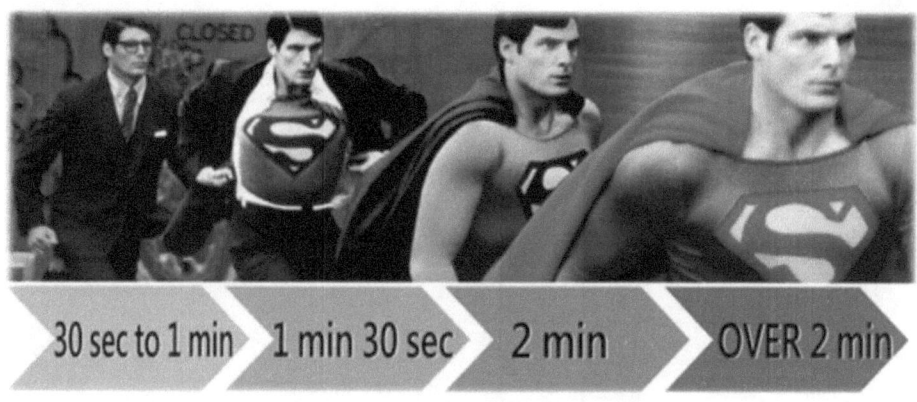

30 sec to 1 min   1 min 30 sec   2 min   OVER 2 min

(Try to break your own breath holding record.)

The average person's breath holding time is about **30 seconds to 1 minute**, which is normal in this range, but if it is less than 30 seconds, it means the lungs capacity is too low, quit smoking quickly, do a health check to prevent the risk of COPD.

If you can hold your breath for more than **a minute**, it means that you are in regular exercise, cardiopulmonary function and physical condition are good, through Eliminate Cravings Breathing Method, as well as maintaining the original regular exercise, and you will be able to quickly eliminate the cravings of cigarettes.

If you can hold your breath for over **1 minute and 30 seconds**, that means your vital capacity and blood oxygen are adequate, you are so strong even you are still smoking. If you can quit smoking, that will make your body function 20 years younger.

If you can hold your breath for **over two minutes**, it really makes me wonder: Are you a human being? You can hold for such a long time of not breathing oxygen, nothing is more difficult than that. Quitting smoking is absolutely not a problem. I believe you can quit smoking smoothly.

Part 2 QUIZ

1. Who is the biggest beneficiary behind cigarettes?
   a. Tobacco farmers
   b. Cigarette manufacturers
   c. The government

2. The author strongly opposes quit smoking by using nicotine products, e-cigarettes, or reducing the amount of smoking... What is the reason?
   a. Too wasteful
   b. It takes too long
   c. All contain nicotine, they are hard to quit

3. When nicotine withdrawal occurs, it will cause headaches, anxiety, irritability, etc., what method should be used to make the withdrawal symptoms disappear?

4. What should you do when a psychological craving occurs?

• Part 3 •

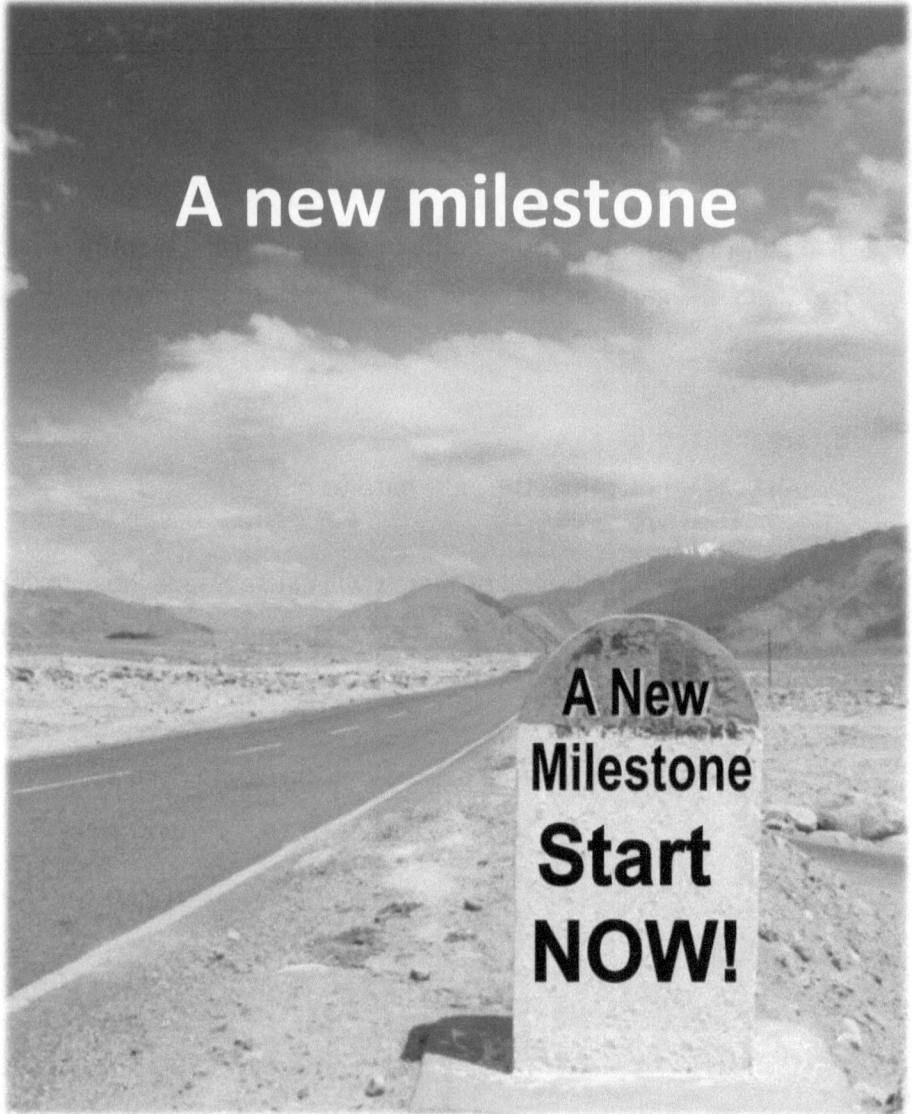

A new milestone

A New
Milestone
Start
NOW!

A new milestone: Today's date
_____ (YYYY-MM-DD),
I started to quit smoking!

Almost everyone who succeeds in quitting smoking remembers exactly when he started. I often feel that quitting smoking is very similar to love, and I often use love as a metaphor for quitting smoking. If you continue the smoking cessation you have done for 30 minutes and decided to quit smoking today, congratulations, and today is a memorable day, just like your wedding anniversary.

Let's take a look at the wedding vow that the priest will read during a wedding: "Will you have this woman to be your wife, to live together in holy marriage and love her, comfort her, honor, and keep her in sickness and in health, and forsaking all others, be faithful to her as long as you both shall live?"

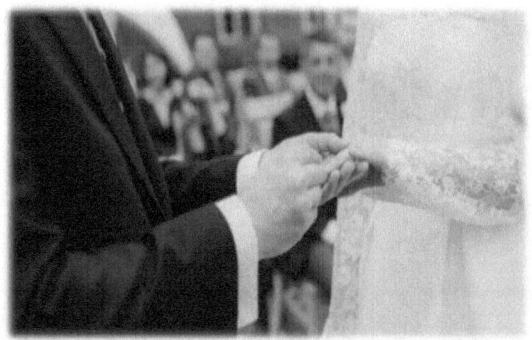

(Think your smoking cessation as you're dealing with your daily marriage life, you will succeed.)

If you are a married person from today, what you should do is how to maintain your marriage, rather than thinking about who you have an ambiguous relationship with, right?

Similarly, if today is the day when you quit smoking, what you should do from now on is to tell yourself that you can't smoke anyway: no matter whether you are still addicted to smoking or not, you can't smoke a cigarette or try a puff to test if your addiction has faded; Not to mention that you can't think of smoking occasionally after the addiction is gone, so you won't worry about getting addicted again.

Once you start smoking again, even if it's just a puff, wouldn't it be similar to a married person had a one-night stand with a stranger? Is it still faithful to marriage?

Many people, after quitting smoking for many years, began to smoke again, not because he faced things bothered him, nor he intentionally wanted to smoke, simply because he was boring, wanted to have fun.

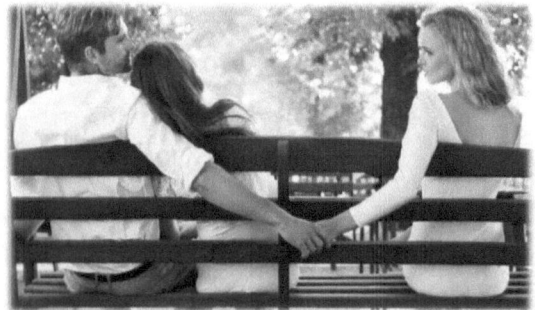

(Don't let cigarettes play a part in your life, or they will be like the affair which will destroy your marriage.)

Like many people who have

affairs, they don't really want to be unfaithful to their partner. Maybe it's just fun at first, but the following things are totally unexpected. Finally, when facing the result of family breakdown, everyone regrets it.

Since you have decided to quit smoking, from now on, cigarettes will be the enemy to your life, just like the extramarital affair which will destroy your marriage. No matter when and where you should always be wary of it inadvertently appearance.

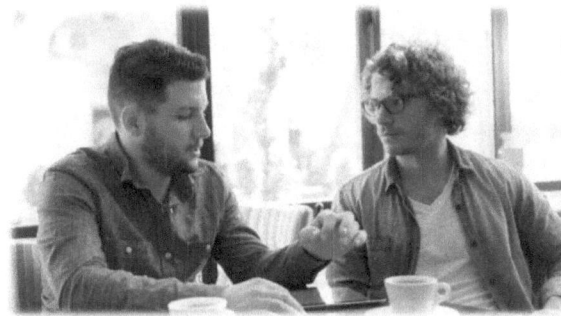

(Find someone who would listen to you, this will play a major role in your smoking cessation.)

Find someone you are close to and trust, share your plan and determination to quit smoking to him/her, and tell him/her:

"I am going to quit smoking. Because you are the most important person to me, so I want to share my decision to quit smoking with you. I will insist on not smoking, even if the cravings are very painful, I will refrain from smoking. I hope you would encourage me during the process, after all, your encouragement is the most powerful motivation for me to keep on quitting smoking.

However, during the process of quitting smoking or in the future, if I want to smoke, I will tell you, but please don't laugh at me or blame me instead remind me, let me recall the deciding scenes in front of you which are happening now. Tell me to cherish the results of non-smoking hours that I have accumulated hard, don't start all over again because I can't stand for the temporary craving.

In case I fail to quit smoking this time, please do not censure me. For me, your silence is already the most severe criticism. Of course, that is the worst situation, I will try my best not to let it happen."

(Your oxygen levels in your blood are increasing now. This helps your muscles become stronger and healthier.)

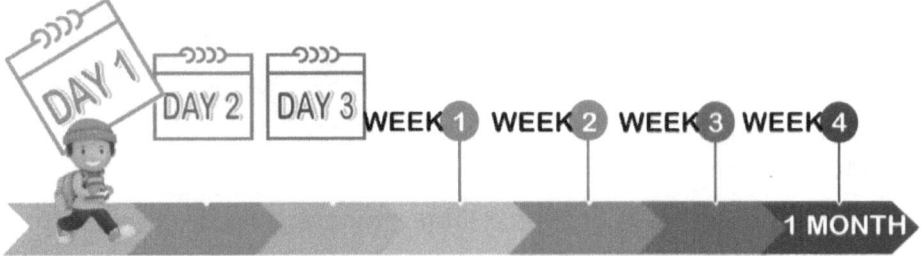

The first stage,

smoking cessation Day 1 ~ Day 3: Day 1

Most people fail to quit smoking during these three days. As long as you can survive these three days without being defeated by tobacco addiction, your chances of success in quitting smoking will increase dramatically to 67%.

The first day of smoking cessation should be fairly easy. The brain seems to be in a state of patience. It's like taking an international flight across continents for more than a dozen hours without smoking, most people can put up with it. Few smokers couldn't stand cravings, would rather risk being punished and go to the toilet on the plane to smoke.

You can take this opportunity to review your situation, which you could not do before when you used to smoke. Because once you thought about cigarettes, you would immediately pick up one to smoke. You never had a chance to stop and observe yourself, to find out what symptoms of withdrawal you have.

A. I feel unwell and depressed.
B. There is no obvious uncomfortable situation, just simply want to smoke.

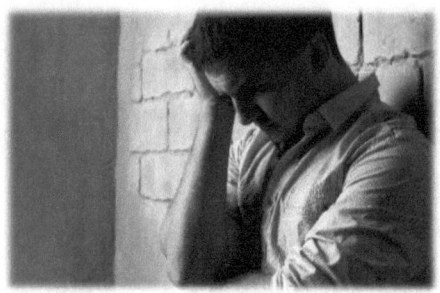

(The withdrawal symptoms usually only last a few minutes, some people won't even feel them, ignore it.)

If it's A, it's the standard nicotine withdrawal symptoms, which produce physiological symptoms called physical addiction. Physical addiction is that your body asks you for cigarettes and tells you to ingest nicotine. It will become milder and milder over time, and the frequency of attacks will be less and less; Physical addiction does not automatically disappear. Before it disappears, you have to show determination and perseverance, tell your body who the boss is, and clearly tell your brain: Don't be led by cigarettes. Of course, it is useless to say it to your brain. As long as you don't buy, don't smoke, don't even think about cigarettes, your body will know it soon, and will make adjustments.

More trouble is B, just simply want to smoke. This is a psychological addiction, and it's easy to be aroused by things around you, called Triggers. Triggers are the things that make you want to smoke. Different people have different triggers, like a stressful situation, sipping coffee, going to a party, or smelling cigarette smoke.

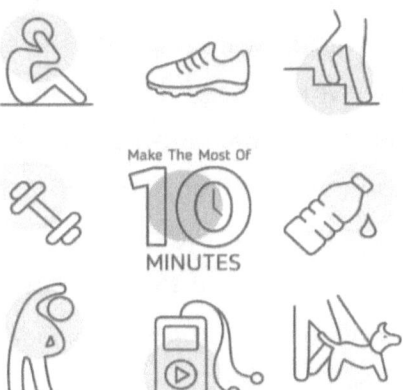

(Besides Eliminate Cravings Breathing, try getting moving, even for just a few minutes, to get through a craving.)

Psychological addiction is difficult to eliminate completely because it is entangled with memories, and you don't know when it will appear, because it may appear with memories. Some people have even quit smoking for more than ten years, psychological addiction would still run out. In my case, the most common psychological addiction after I quit smoking is dreaming of smoking. To tell you the truth, smoking in dreams feels real and cool. I often dreamed smoking during the first two years of quitting smoking, sometimes it still happens.

Whether it is a physical craving or a psychological addiction, at least you start to recognize the appearance of cigarettes. This is a crucial step in overcoming addiction. You can feel when the addiction attacks and how it exists, then you can find a way to get rid of it.

When you are determined to start smoking cessation, you can use the weekend as the day to start smoking cessation. Generally speaking, the most difficult thing to conquer during the period of smoking cessation is the discomfort caused by withdrawal symptoms. If you smoked a pack of cigarettes a day, the symptoms of the discomfort will occur about 20 times a day, which means the withdrawal symptoms will occur every half an hour, and each episode will last about 3 to 5 minutes. The most intense attack of withdrawal symptoms will fall on the second to the third day of smoking cessation, then the times of attack slowly decrease as the number of days of smoking cessation increase.

Some people go through the first three days by sleeping and taking a cold shower, that's because they don't know Eliminate Cravings Breathing Method. Never underestimate the breathing method, this is a weapon against the symptoms of withdrawal, specifically to deal with physiological addiction, must make good use of it, as soon as the withdrawal symptoms appear, use it right away, don't hesitate, withdrawal symptoms will be relieved immediately.

Besides Eliminate Cravings Breathing Method, you can drink more water, do some exercises that make you sweat, and do things that you can divert your attention. One thing to remember is that the body's withdrawal symptoms are stronger in the first three days, but they are absolutely bearable, and they are weakened day after day. Every time you experience a withdrawal symptom, you are one step closer to completely breaking away from cigarette addiction.

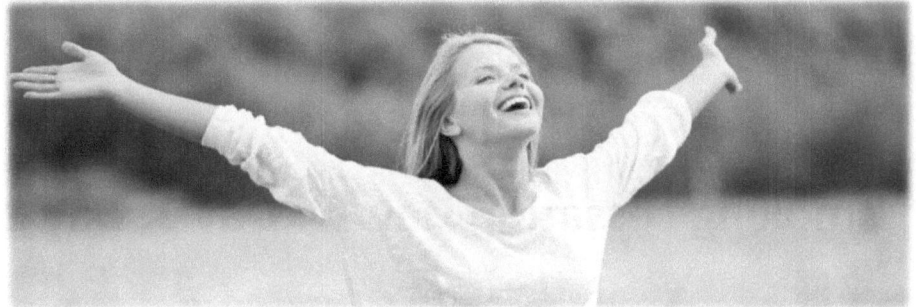

(Soon you will feel the real freedom.)

(Free yourself. Quitting means never worrying about where your next pack of cigarettes is coming from.)

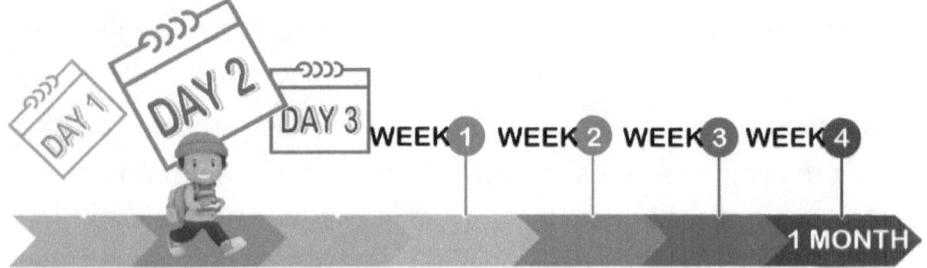

The first stage,

smoking cessation Day 1 ~ Day 3: Day 2

Most people feel that the second day of smoking cessation is the most difficult time to get through.

According to the opinions of smokers and my personal experience, most people give up their smoking cessation on this day. The brain no longer sleeps, it wakes up and desperately asks for cigarettes, regardless of physical or psychological addiction, all are attacking.

This is the day that the willpower of quitting smoking is facing the greatest challenge. A lot of thoughts come up in your head, just like someone is whispering into your ear: "Quit smoking another day, It's OK to take a puff, or use a nicotine patch..."

You will have a feeling that quitting smoking is like an endless road, it is so tired that it's useless to quit. Why hasn't the addiction disappeared? When will the addiction vanish? Isn't it true that the addiction will always exist?

Actually, such a feeling will appear again and again. This is just one of the physical symptoms of nicotine withdrawal. It usually appears for a few minutes and then disappears. And the frequency of appearance will be less and less, don't be fooled by this feeling, and smoke a cigarette or use nicotine products. Otherwise, the road to successfully quit smoking will never go to the end.

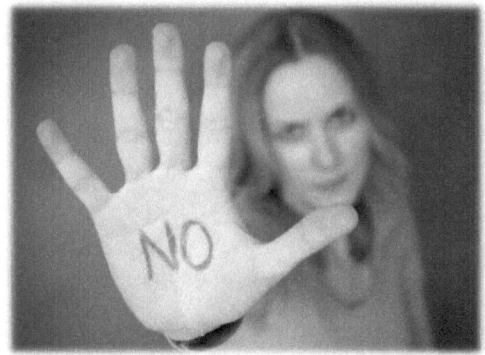

(Say "NO" to those negative thoughts. It's time to tell your brain who the BOSS is.)

The purpose I am telling you these things is because I hope you are prepared, so the cravings won't catch you off guard. I want you to know that these symptoms will occur, and also they will soon disappear. Don't shake your will to quit smoking because of the symptoms. "No matter how I quit is useless." This is the most common thought that always comes to smokers mind when failing to quit smoking. Don't let it beat you.

Smoking addiction, like the devil, it gives the brain an illusion that quitting smoking is impossible to succeed, so you can't persist in. But in fact, the real quitting begins when the symptoms of withdrawal appear, it is also the beginning of the challenge for a smoker to demonstrate his determination to the devil.

Please remember to use Eliminate Cravings Breathing Method, which can quickly remove the discomfort caused by cigarette addiction. When you breathe with Eliminate Cravings Breathing Method, your body will be in a state of pseudo-hypoxia, which makes your brain think that you are in an oxygen-deficient environment and you are in danger. When the brain thinks that the body is hypoxic, it orders the body to breathe oxygen as a priority, not smoking, and it also suspends everything related to cigarettes or cigarette addiction.

It's like a drowning man who cries for help in the water and he is sinking. At this time you throw a cigarette, and a can of oxygen, which one do you think he wants? He, of course, grabbed the oxygen cylinder immediately. In the subconscious mind of the brain, it is very clear that cigarettes are not necessary to maintain life. When cigarettes are in contact with the survival of life, cigarettes will be immediately put aside. The brain will wait for safety, then continue to ask cigarettes from you.

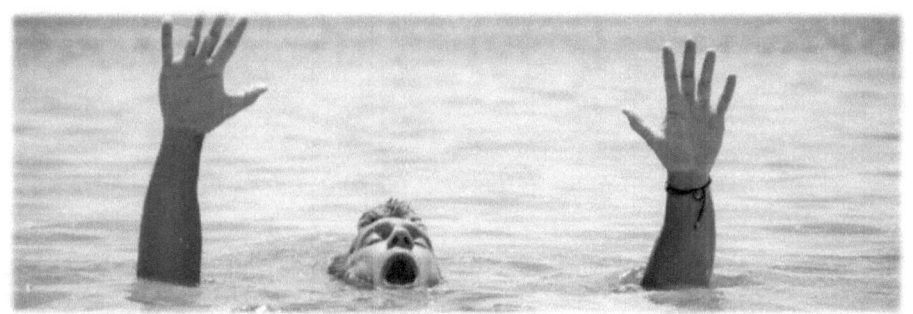

(Cheat your brain with Eliminate Cravings Breathing.)

After starting to quit smoking, if you pay close attention to your situation, you will find: Usually, your body is under your control and coordinates well. But when you quit smoking, there is a conflict between your body and your consciousness. Then your body becomes disobedient and seems to be another person. These phenomena are very interesting. The feedback of withdrawal symptoms through smoking cessation can be strictly subdivided into: physical, psychological, and conscious, that is, body, mind, and spirit. You will find that the contradictions and conflicts caused by quitting smoking make the three parts of the body, mind, and spirit produce different expressions. If you can observe such a situation, this will help you to know yourself more deeply and feel what is the existence of "true you".

(Free yourself. Quitting means never worrying about where your next pack of cigarettes is coming from.)

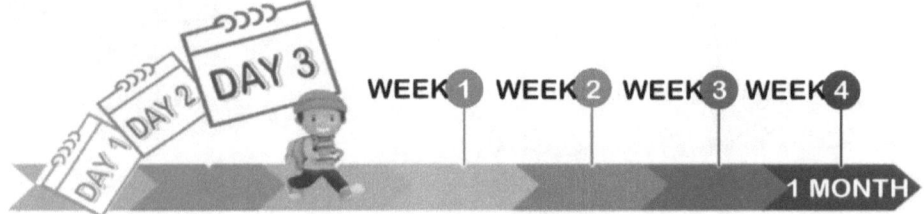

The first stage,
smoking cessation Day 1 ~ Day 3: Day 3

After the suffering of the previous day, you entered the third day of smoking cessation. If you're still quitting smoking so far, then I have to say you're a warrior. Two-thirds of people in the world who quit smoking can't last three days, but it seems you not only can survive today, but you certainly can last for a week. It is so obvious that you have found a way to quit smoking, adjust yourself to the best condition.

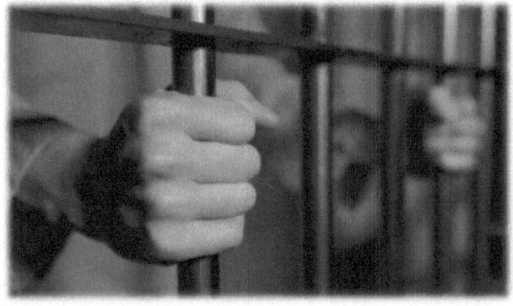

(Over 90% of smokers are trapped over 30 years. This is longer than the time that most prisoners who were sentenced to jail.)

After the twists and tosses of the second day, I can tell you with certainty that there will be no worse withdrawal symptoms like yesterday in your future smoking cessation. But that doesn't mean you've got rid of your addiction ever since. You still have a way to go, but the worst situation is over.

More than 90% of people, the strongest withdrawal symptoms appear on the second smoking cessation day. But there are a small number of people whose most uncomfortable withdrawal symptoms appear later, about the third to fifth days. The reason why this happens is unknown. Probably because these people smoke less than others, so the density of nicotine in their bodies are low, and the brains respond slowly to the lack of nicotine.

On the third day, the symptoms of addiction withdrawal are still uncomfortable, the level of discomfort may be not dropping, but the times of addiction attack are significantly reduced. You would still feel withdrawal symptoms and psychological addiction at the original cigarettes smoked when you do certain things, such as after meals, talking, getting up ..., besides that, those cigarettes that were not meant to smoke would become less likely to smoke. For example, you go jogging every day, and sometimes you smoke a cigarette while taking a break. But on the third day of quitting smoking, you would obviously feel no need for smoking the cigarette at a non-specific time, and some people may even reject it.

Being able to stop smoking for more than 48 hours is something you haven't done before. A firm mind is the key to your success in quitting smoking. Occasionally, even if your mind is not strong enough, pull yourself back to your original intention. The reason that makes you quit smoking at the beginning is the greatest motivation for you to carry out the whole smoking cessation program.

The body's withdrawal response will become milder and milder. It would be a great pity for you to give up the cessation hours that you have already accumulated if you can't stand the current uncomfortable feelings. Unless you will never quit smoking, or you will have to go through the same things again on the next time. How painful it is! The most uncomfortable part has passed, and the rest is keeping in the present state.

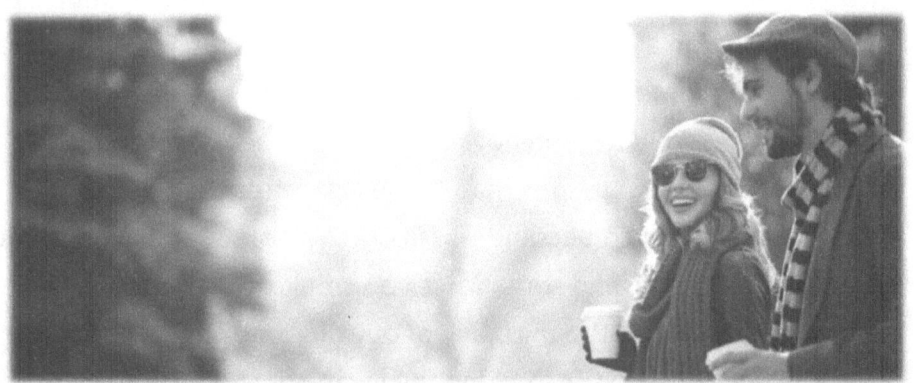

(Craving a smoke? Talk to a friend! You don't have to do this alone.)

But I must remind you again and again that the psychological addiction may be repeated from time to time. Even after many years of smoking cessation, sometimes there is still the urge to smoke. This kind of psychological addiction will not cause any pain to you. Usually, if you ignore it, it will disappear within a minute. But if you put it into action, pick up a cigarette and take a puff, then you will fall back into the original trap cycle.

Remember, cigarettes are your eternal enemy. The cigarette itself may not be guilty, but the diseases that accompany it, as well as the huge profits behind it, are all caused by cigarettes.

If you are suffering, uncomfortable and depressed now, you should know that these symptoms of discomfort are not what you were born with, nor what this book brought to you, but cigarettes.

To fight against psychological addiction, you should repeatedly ask yourself the following questions, even if you already know the answer:

What is the reason I am determined to quit smoking?
What are the benefits of smoking?
Do I really like smoking?

(Certain places can be a trigger to smoke. Be careful when you're there.)

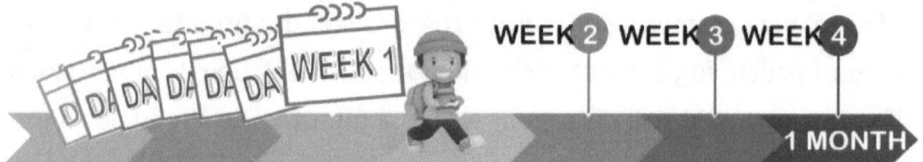

The second stage,

smoking cessation Day 4 ~ Day 7: Week 1

You are awesome, successfully spent the three days of the most difficult time in the smoking cessation process. Let's greet the second stage together and challenge smoking cessation for a week.

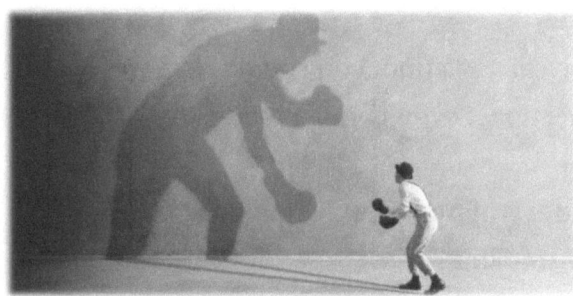

(Exercise boosts your endorphins, gives you time to clear your head, and makes you feel great.)

According to statistics, if you can hold on for another four days, that is, when you quit smoking for seven days, at the end of the second stage, your success rate of quitting smoking will be as high as 95%. In other words, most people have given up before they have reached your record. And only 5 percent of people who quit smoking can achieve the same status as you. Obviously, you are more determination and perseverance than others. I believe your family must be very proud of you.

I believe you already know how to use Eliminate Cravings Breathing Method to overcome the withdrawal symptoms of cigarette addiction attacks. You must have discovered the withdrawal symptoms that were originally annoying to you are becoming minor and the frequency of withdrawal is gradually decreasing. Almost all the time you would have smoked and the things you would have done while smoking had to be at least once. Almost everything you would have smoked, and what you would do while smoking, have to go through at least one round, and before the addiction disappeared, you have not smoked or used nicotine-related products, then your brain will accept the fact that there is no nicotine or cigarettes at a specific time or the special things.

Do you understand my explanation? At the present stage, you have experienced most of the things in a smokeless state, including all the routines in life, such as getting up, eating, sleeping, going to the toilet, etc. You have spent without cigarettes. The more these routines happen over time, the less the brain will ask for cigarettes from you. But you have to be wary of things that you don't do every day. Let's say you used to play cards at a friend's house once a week. On that occasion, everyone was smoking, and you smoked a lot of cigarettes. If you play cards again, your friends will certainly advise you to smoke, you will also because you did not quit smoking yet when playing cards last time, so that the brain's memory part and the craving part will link together, causes the desire to smoke.

There are many other things like this. Sometimes it is not certainly a "THING", like re-visiting old places may also arouse the connection between cravings and memories. But as long as you pay attention, these sudden feelings are hard to beat you. After all, the most uncomfortable you have experienced, and the following withdrawal of the physiological addiction will only become lighter and lighter, the frequency of psychological addiction will also decrease. As long as you are on guard against cigarettes and avoid accidentally arousing interest in them, your smoking cessation will go very smoothly.

(Even one cig will make it hard to stay SmokeFree.)

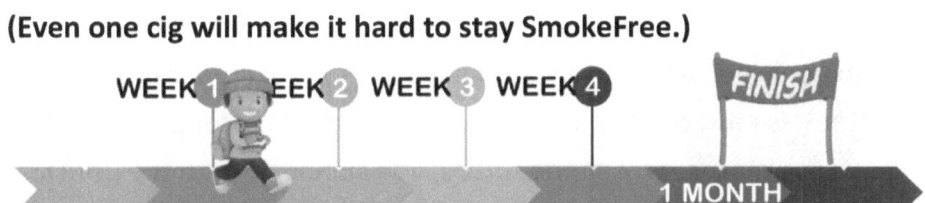

The third stage,

smoking cessation Week 2 ~ Week 4:

Month 1

The third stage, which is about to enter, is the final stage of smoking cessation in this book, but it does not mean the end of smoking cessation, but you have good knowledge, determination, and perseverance in quit smoking. Your achievement in quitting smoking is a good example for others because only one percent of people can complete this stage; in other words, when you complete this smoking cessation stage, your success rate of quitting smoking will reach 99%, equivalent to the success of quitting smoking.

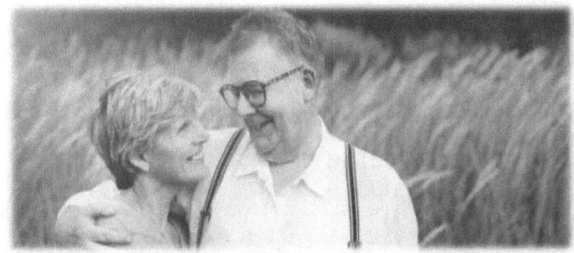

(Quitting smoking is hard. It's a process that may take time, but it can be just as tough to stay smokefree.)

Is it difficult to quit smoking, or is it easy? The answer to this question, maybe only you are the most qualified person to answer it. But no matter it is hard or easy, I believe you want to go through that again. That's the reason why, in the future, you should stick to the principles of not puffing, not touching or even thinking of cigarettes. If you have any of these thoughts, it means that there still are cravings inside your mind. You must completely clean them all out.

Have you cleaned up your cigarette addiction? You can tell it from whether you want to smoke a cigarette to test it. For example, a prisoner who is imprisoned is always eager for freedom and thinking about freedom because he is behind the bars. But a free man does not think whether he is in a free environment, nor does he need to experience the feeling of freedom through being kept in prison, or to test the existence of freedom through imprisonment.

Please don't think I'm forbidding you to smoke, even if you don't even think about it. I remind you again and again that all the failures in quitting smoking are due to the lack of precaution against cigarettes after quitting smoking for a while and then try again.

Remember, not even a puff!

"Just take a puff." When this idea comes out, it's a wildfire of thought. Put it out right away and it will start a prairie fire.

"Just take a puff." It was just a puff of cigarettes that caused you to work so hard to give up smoking now.

"Just take a puff and help me get through the difficulties I am facing now, then I'll quit smoking later." Such an idea will disintegrate all efforts, and everything will have to be done again.

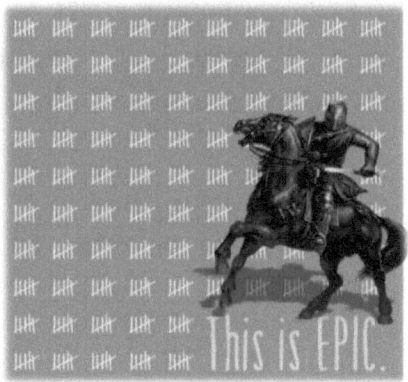

(This won't be easy or quick. It will be every day, and each day you will emerge a victor... your own hero. This is epic.)

Some people think that taking a puff is just to make sure that he no longer needs cigarettes, and only a puff, that's all. Some people think that cigarettes taste terrible after taking a puff. The smoker thinks that he will never be attracted again, but what he did was attracted again. When smokers finally break the chain of cigarette addiction, it takes only a puff, a cigarette, and they will be sent back to the original trap.

Sometimes you will think that this is a tug-of-war between you and the end of the cigarette addiction. But the truth is, every time you feel this way, you're close enough to say goodbye to the addiction.

People who quit smoking usually can feel that "smoking addiction is gone" before the end of this stage. It's a moment of freedom. It's as if it's sunny after the rain. You'll realize that you're completely free from the addiction, you can go anywhere without anxiety, there is no need to worry about the problem of smoking areas. From this moment on, all the commercial, brainwashing, and traditional cigarette image advertisements and publicity effects have all disappeared. When you see other smokers on the road, you will feel that you are better than them.

Such feelings, including the disappearance of smoking addiction, the superiority of smoking cessation success, are due to you have established a "disgust" for cigarettes before starting to quit smoking. Only when we really hate cigarettes from the heart can we permanently eliminate psychological addiction. Because the motivation to quit smoking comes from the dislike of cigarettes, when the addiction to cigarettes is eliminated, it will immediately feel that it is no longer bound.

If you are in a way of forbearance and repression from the beginning, not because you have seen through the intrigue of cigarettes, expecting that you will quit successfully if you endure long enough, or during the cessation, you still smoke or use nicotine substitutes, then it is recommended that you start from the beginning, figure out the essence of the "you want to smoke" first, follow the steps in the book, and you will achieve the goal of completely quitting smoking, too.

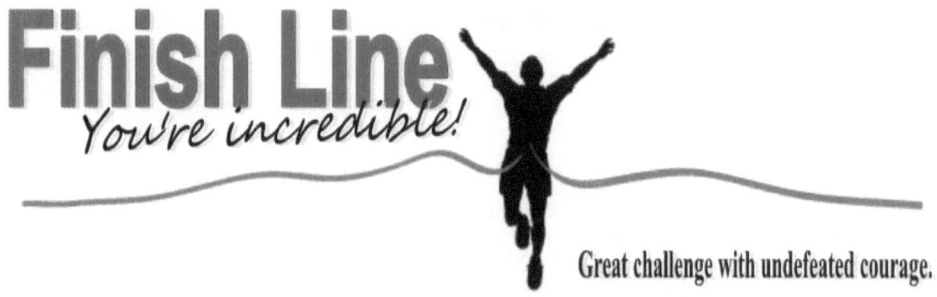

Finish Line

You're incredible!

Great challenge with undefeated courage.

Congratulations on completing the third stage of quitting smoking. Now you can tell everyone loudly: Yeah, I am a non-smoking person.

In fact, you may feel that you have already got rid of the addiction as early as two weeks ago, but you probably weren't quite sure how successful you were in quitting smoking. Now, you not only have no desire to smoke, but you can also share your smoking cessation experience with others.

As long as the smokers fully follow the cessation rules, quitting smoking will success:

◎ **Find someone you trust and tell him your determination to quit smoking. Ask him to encourage you in the process of quitting**

smoking.

It is important to speak out your determination to quit smoking and the mood in the process of quitting smoking. The object whom you declare your determination to can be a person or a group, but the premise must be: This is someone your trust, and if you fail to quit, he will not ridicule or satirize you so that you can face him honestly.

Please share the quitting methods and specifications that you have learned in this book with the person who is gonna help you quit smoking so he will know what to do to help you correctly and remind you at the right time, instead of just telling you "Hang in there." or ask you to quit smoking in the wrong way.

◎ **You won't lose or give up anything, because cigarettes won't give you any enjoyment, and all the fun and pleasure you get from smoking is something you can get through other things.**

Please don't think that I keep reiterating that it will be better after quitting smoking which is meant to brainwash you or I am an outsider, I can't understand why everyone smokes. If it is not because you also agree, that quitting smoking is better, I don't think you would have read this chapter from the front page of the book. All the pleasures and fun are actually built on the addiction to nicotine and the illusion. Once you get rid of the addiction, you can easily get the pleasure of being deprived back.

◎ **The most uncomfortable period from the first three days to the first week of smoking cessation, you should do Eliminate Cravings Breathing Method and repeatedly ask yourself the three core questions of quitting smoking.**

Don't let the discomfort during the withdrawal process interrupt your smoking cessation program. Everything you have experienced is exactly the same thing that millions of other people have experienced. The most effective way to solve the physical and psychological withdrawal symptoms at the same time is self-question three core questions of quitting smoking and do Eliminate Cravings Breathing Method.

◎ **Do not use any substitute to quit smoking.**

Any nicotine product or use any other things to help you quit smoking will only make quitting more difficult and easier to relapse.

◎ **Don't be deceived by insecurity, and don't worry about when the addiction will go away, just focus on your original life.**

When you start to quit smoking, it's normal to feel apprehensive without cigarettes. This is the uneasiness caused by the cravings.

As long as you stick to the belief of quitting smoking, ignore it and do not feed the addiction, it will soon disappear. When the uneasiness disappears, you will feel the real freedom, which is the addiction completely dissipates.

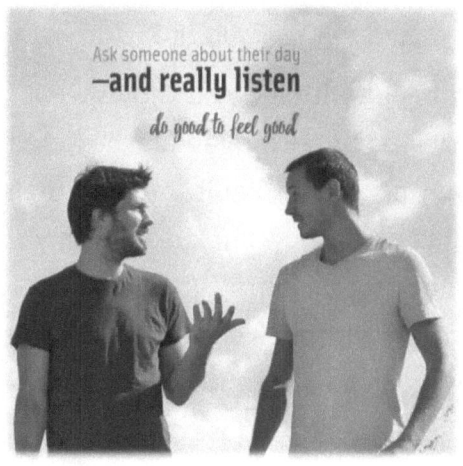

(Do good to feel good. Being kind to others lifts you both up, which can be helpful during your quit.)

Think about it. If your friends and relatives around you who are suffering from cigarette addiction and notice that you have quit smoking successfully, ask you how to quit smoking. What do you think is the first step to quit smoking?

The reason I ask this is smoking is declining rapidly. If you smoke for more than ten years, you will definitely feel that smoking is becoming more and more unpopular, that the price of cigarettes is getting higher and higher, and there are fewer and fewer occasions allow smoking.

As smokers are excluded, more people quit smoking, and the remaining smokers become lonelier. They also have to spend more money on cigarettes, all they get is the inhalation of nicotine, and carcinogenic tar and chemicals.

A smoker is also aware of the situation he is facing. You don't need to emphasize the disadvantages of smoking with him, he knows what will eventually happen. There is no need to tell him about the benefits of quitting smoking, because he may not want to quit smoking at all, continuous emphasis on the benefits of quitting smoking will only increase his annoyance. You only need to tell him: "Why not test yourself and see how long you can stay without a cigarette. Just try it anyway, if you can't stand the cravings, you can continue to smoke, that's the worst situation, and there is nothing to lose." If he feels interested, then share your quitting experience with him. Otherwise, it will only increase his dislike for quitting smoking.

(About 40 percent of smokers who quit say that support from others mattered a lot in their success.)

If you are afraid that you can't fully express your smoking cessation method, then recommend this book to him. This book can help him quit cigarettes at a cost of less than a pack of cigarettes. If he would rather spend money on buying cigarettes than this book, that means his intention to quit smoking may not be strong enough, then why persuade him to quit smoking?

You can quit smoking successfully, the greatest achievement is not this book, but you.
You can quit smoking successfully, the hardest part is not just to quit smoking, but you are willing to do so.
You can quit smoking successfully, the most admirable thing is not that you can resist, but that you can persist.